Shelter and Service Issues for Aging Populations: International Perspectives

Shelter and Service Issues for Aging Populations: International Perspectives

Leon A. Pastalan
Editor

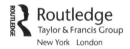

Routledge
Taylor & Francis Group
New York   London

First published 1997 by The Haworth Press, Inc.

This edition published 2013 by Routledge

711 Third Avenue, New York, NY 10017
2 Park Square, Milton Park, Abingdon, Oxon OX14 4RN

Routledge is an imprint of the Taylor & Francis Group, an informa business

Shelter and Service Issues for Aging Populations: International Perspectives has also been published as *Journal of Housing for the Elderly*, Volume 12, Numbers 1/2 1997.

The development, preparation, and publication of this work has been undertaken with great care. However, the publisher, employees, editors, and agents of The Haworth Press and all imprints of The Haworth Press, Inc., including The Haworth Medical Press and Pharmaceutical Products Press, are not responsible for any errors contained herein or for consequences that may ensue from use of materials or information contained in this work. Opinions expressed by the author(s) are not necessarily those of The Haworth Press, Inc.

Cover design by Thomas J. Mayshock Jr.

Library of Congress Cataloging-in-Publication Data

Shelter and service issues for aging populations : international perspectives / Leon A. Pastalan, editor.
    p. cm.
    Published also as Vol. 12, Nos. 1-2 of Journal of housing for the elderly.
    Includes bibliographical references and index.
    ISBN 0-7890-0314-7 (alk. paper). – ISBN 0-7890-1330-4 (pbk.)
    1. Aged–Housing–United States. 2. Aged–Housing–Europe, Western. 3. Aged–Housing–United States–Planning. 4. Aged–Housing–Europe, Western–Planning. 5. Aged–Services for–United States. 6. Aged–Services for–Europe, Western. I. Pastalan, Leon A., 1930- .
HD7287.92.U54S47 1997   97-16059
362.6'3'094–dc21   CIP

Shelter and Service Issues for Aging Populations: International Perspectives

CONTENTS

ABOUT THE EDITOR

Leon A. Pastalan, PhD, is Professor of Architecture in the College of Architecture and Urban Planning at The University of Michigan. Dr. Pastalan is also Director of the National Center on Housing and Living Arrangements for Older Americans. As a researcher of long standing in the field of environments for the elderly, he is an expert in sensory deficits, spatial behavior, and housing. Dr. Pastalan has published many books and articles resulting from his work, including *Man Environment Reference 2* (MER 2) (The University of Michigan Press, 1983), *Retirement Communities: An American Original* (The Haworth Press, Inc., 1984), *Lifestyles and Housing of Older Adults: The Florida Experience* (The Haworth Press, Inc., 1989), *Aging in Place: The Role of Housing and Social Supports* (The Haworth Press, Inc., 1990), *Optimizing Housing for the Elderly: Homes Not Houses* (The Haworth Press, Inc., 1991) and most recently, *University-Linked Retirement Communities: Student Visions of Eldercare* (The Haworth Press, Inc., 1994) and *Housing Decisions for the Elderly: To Move or Not to Move* (The Haworth Press, Inc., 1995). Dr. Pastalan is also Editor of the *Journal of Housing for the Elderly* (The Haworth Press, Inc.).

Chapter 1

An Introduction
to International Perspectives
on Shelter and Service Issues
for Aging Populations

Leon A. Pastalan

INTRODUCTION

This volume is devoted to an international perspective. Due to cultural and historical factors, the focus is on the experiences of countries in Western Europe and North America. It is hoped that future publications will be able to print the accounts of countries from other parts of the World in terms of how they dealt with housing and service needs of their elders.

Western Europe and North America, despite the many options and/or alternatives in addressing housing and service issues for the elderly, essentially reflect only two basic approaches, that of (1) the provision of specialized facilities through purposeful design, construction and operation or (2) provision of support services as a way of dealing with changing needs and maintaining people in the community.

Leon A. Pastalan, PhD, is affiliated with the College of Architecture and Urban Planning, 2225A Art and Architecture Building, The University of Michigan, Ann Arbor, MI 48109-2069.

[Haworth co-indexing entry note]: "An Introduction to International Perspectives on Shelter and Service Issues for Aging Populations." Pastalan, Leon A. Co-published simultaneously in *Journal of Housing for the Elderly* (The Haworth Press, Inc.) Vol. 12, No. 1/2, 1997, pp. 1-7; and: *Shelter and Service Issues for Aging Populations: International Perspectives* (ed: Leon A. Pastalan) The Haworth Press, Inc., 1997, pp. 1-7. Single or multiple copies of this article are available for a fee from The Haworth Document Delivery Service [1-800-342-9678, 9:00 a.m. - 5:00 p.m. (EST). E-mail address: getinfo@ haworth.com].

The experience over the past thirty years or so has been to emphasize one approach or the other and at times both simultaneously. The 1960's and 1970's, for instance, witnessed a great deal of specialized facilities being constructed and operated. The Scandinavian countries led the way with this approach. Sweden, for instance, built approximately one million units of such specialized housing. France, The Netherlands, Britain, the United States, Canada and other Western countries were also part of this movement.

Specialized housing facilities had a number of very positive features such as concentrations of people to provide a critical mass for service delivery; a concentrated number of residents that were proximitous and easily accessible for friendship formation and social support to replace friends and significant others lost through illness and death; provided persons with limited incomes access to quality housing and created many opportunities for public and private agencies and organizations to test develop models regarding design requirements, construction techniques, building types, service delivery systems and management philosophies. The negative side of this approach was the high cost of such facilities in terms of construction and maintenance, failure to anticipate increased need for support services as resident populations aged and the inability of most countries economically to build enough units to satisfy the demand for such housing. Nonetheless, this was a period of great optimism, exper-imentation and learning.

The late 1970's and the 1980's was a period of reduced construction of specialized facilities and the beginning of the search for alternatives. A number of Western European countries expanded their community-based support services as a way of responding to changing functional and finan-cial needs and to maintain older residents in their homes and delaying the onset of institutionalization. This was a time, particularly in Europe, where the shift away from constructing specialized facilities as a way of solving shelter and service needs to one where community support services be-came the accepted approach.

The North American trend in the 1980's seemed to be split between efforts to continue the construction of specialized facilities while at the same time initiating the development of community support services. The Canadian effort, for example, continued to build new facilities and at the same time was developing community-based support services which were largely financed with public funds. In the United States meanwhile, the 1980's reflected the Reagan Era where the Federal presence regarding publicly financed housing programs for the elderly virtually disappeared and community-based services were struggling in terms of their development due to the general unavailability of funding. While the public sector was decimated, the private sector was busily engaged in the development of CCRCs and other types of retirement communities that responded to shelter and service needs ranging from residential to health care. To be sure, these efforts were largely focused on the middle class who could afford to live in such facilities. The 1990's is witnessing the predominance of community-based services in contrast to specially designed facilities as the preferred solution to shelter and service needs of older people. While this movement had been going on for quite some time in Western Europe and Canada, the Americans were late in coming to this approach but sometime in the late 1980's politicians, public officials and a variety of others discovered something called "aging in place" and it has become something of a national mantra. It seems everyone is in favor of "aging in place" even though there is only a vague idea of what this concept actually means in practical or policy terms. Politicians and public officials are attracted to it because they view it as less costly than other alternatives; service providers like it because they can serve larger numbers of people and older people like it because they think it means there is now a mechanism to help them remain in their present residential circumstances.

Contributors to this volume help to clarify some of the issues mentioned above and add very valuable new data and insights to the shelter and service challenges the West has been grappling with for a long time. Wister and Gutman, for instance, present an historical overview of 30 years of housing programs in Canada along with a discussion of emerging trends in meeting the housing needs of older Canadians. Their perceptive review of housing philosophies that characterized Canadian policies and programs paralleled the experiences of most Western countries. The authors point out what seems to be a universal problem and that is the lack of coordination of services and shelter in a way that responds to a continuum of changes in the individual. This lack is said to be in part due to the inability of many elders to anticipate and respond appropriately to change in function. There is the issue of people remaining in the community too long which calls attention to the limits of an "aging in place" philosophy. This is an issue that will no doubt become an increasingly important one, particularly in North America as experience with this housing alternative begins to sort itself out.

Tinker provides significant information from the United Kingdom regarding housing choices and policies at different stages of middle and old age and on the developing range of housing options to meet these needs. Older people in the UK wish to remain in their own homes as do most people elsewhere in the world. According to Tinker, there are two major housing options available for older British people. One is to stay at home with a package of services and the other is to move to special housing arrangements such as very sheltered housing. Very sheltered housing is described as provision of meals, extra wardens, domiciliary assistants, and additional communal facilities. Britain has experienced a decline in public sector building of small specially designed housing in favor of other alternatives. Finally, there is also a concern that adequate services in the future may become a serious problem as demand will exceed the supply.

The lack of adequate support services for older people throughout Western Europe and North America has a number of causes not the least of which may be a stigma which seems to attend the elderly. There is a feeling on the part of many persons who serve the old, as well as the old themselves, that somehow the public perception tends to be that all old people are poor, sick, helpless and institutionalized. Page conducted a study which seems to suggest that there is more than just a feeling. He found definite stigmatizing effects of the elderly label in efforts to obtain rental housing in two Canadian cities. Rooms were significantly more likely to be described as unavailable when the caller was elderly. It appears that despite increased knowledge regarding the elderly in society, persons identified as elderly still face the prospect of rejection. The author raises a very interesting issue, that of identifying community situations in which the general public's accepting attitudes toward the elderly may not be consistent with its private reactions and behaviors. It would be instructive to do an international study to determine how universal is this problem.

Hallman and Joseph's case study of a well-known English housing model called Abbeyfield focused on how well such a model adapts to the Canadian experience. The Abbeyfield model of congregate housing originated in Britain more than thirty years ago and it is now promoted by an international federation of volunteer-based local societies. The primary objective of each Abbeyfield Society is the provision of family-like accommodation for single elderly people. The essence of the Abbeyfield model, the authors tell us, is that it emphasizes lifestyle as much as shelter. One general conclusion of this study was that the introduction of a new housing alternative was met with some resistance on the part of local elderly residents and public officials alike. The whole spectrum of "change agentry" was at issue here as much as the new housing concept itself. The authors did find that Abbeyfield was an excellent solution for congregate housing needs in small rural communities. It wasn't only the scale and the "home-like" ambience that met with a positive response but also a housing model that responded to the widely dispersed and low numbers of persons living in such communities. As is well-known, providing responsive, high quality housing and living arrangements and other services that are cost effective in rural areas has been a very difficult task and most efforts to date have not been all that successful. Abbeyfield appears to be an exception and the authors feel it deserves a place among the various alternative housing models, particularly as it applies to rural areas.

Dr. Carmon presents a case study of a post-occupancy evaluation of a CCRC (continuing care retirement community) located in Israel. The CCRC model has been a popular housing alternative in the United States for many years. While its popularity is very high in the U.S., it does not seem to be as popular elsewhere in the World. That is why Dr. Carmon's study of a CCRC in Israel is of special interest. The author in the course of her evaluation developed a checklist which she found useful regarding the determination of housing-related needs in terms of the physical-functional and psycho-social dimensions. Perhaps one of the most significant findings in this study was that the residents considered the individual spatial domain to be of utmost importance. If they were satisfied with their personal spatial domain they tended to be satisfied with other areas of the community. While the facility Dr. Carmon described more closely resembled a home for aged in the United States, it nonetheless is instructive to learn about such communities elsewhere.

Barrier-free housing policies as they relate to elderly people is an emerging area of concern internationally. Peter Dunn describes a range of policy options and approaches taken by Canada and the United States including construction, community service programs, building codes and regulations, and human rights legislation. The strengths and weaknesses of these approaches and policies are contrasted. Each country emphasizes a different strategy with the United States focusing on individual housing rights while Canada reflects a more social welfare approach. Dr. Dunn concludes his discourse with offering a possible new model for barrier-free housing policies and outlines the next steps for making the housing environment more responsive to the needs of elderly people with disabilities.

Rural and urban neighborhoods have long been thought to be different from one another in terms of their preferences regarding amenities and services. Zachary Zimmer and Neena Chappell found that when addressing the subject of housing for older adults it is important to consider not only the built environment but the neighborhood surroundings as well. These investigators undertook a study to examine amenity preferences of a sample (N 1,408) of rural and urban elderly Canadians. They found three types of amenities that were important to seniors no matter where they lived. These were: (1) necessities (e.g., food store); (2) social interaction (such as friends and neighbors nearby); and (3) life enrichment (access to library, entertainment, etc.). One of the strongest findings regarding differences between rural and urban elders was that rural residents rated social interaction and necessity items more important than did their urban counterparts. Also, rural residents gave a lower preference to enrichment items than did urban residents. Results of statistical analyses demonstrate the importance of social interaction amenities to rural elders, confirming the instrumental importance that social relations serve for those living in rural areas. It would be useful to do a cross-national study of amenity preferences to determine to what extent the outcomes found in this study apply to other Western countries.

In a different look at neighborhoods, Elia Werczberger examines a number of factors which affect the demographic ecology of urban areas. Specifically, it looks at the effects of demographical aging on the urban ecology, namely the spatial concentration of the elderly. The author used what he calls a "quasi-dynamic" simulation model based on an accounting framework to analyze the combined effects of the aging households and of residential buildings. Three factors were shown to bring about the spatial integration of different age groups: (1) spatial mobility; (2) non-durable housing; and (3) household dissolution. Werczberger concludes that in a growing city, new households concentrate at the periphery creating a gradual outmoving suburban ring of young households. As these neighborhoods become older, an integrated age distribution develops. On the other hand, age-specific preferences regarding the demographic composition of neighborhoods and relocation lead to a lasting spatial concentration of elderly households. The author also discusses implications for future research and limitations of his model.

Regulations of specialized housing for the elderly exist in all industrialized countries. The regulatory climate can have alternatively an enhancing and/or a chilling effect on the quality, quantity and appropriateness of housing for older adults. Professor Alexander undertakes the Herculean task of describing and comparing regulatory systems of Germany, Israel, The Netherlands, the United Kingdom, and the United States. From these comparisons he derives what he considers are elements for an ideal regulatory framework. The author notes that no one regulatory structure or procedure is innately superior and the wide variation between and among countries is less attributable to deliberate design than to historical circumstances. Whatever approach is taken, a balance must be established between a permissive approach which can promote diversity, creativity, and responsiveness to consumer demands, but at the same time, risks abuse on the one hand and an oppressive bureaucracy that limits abuses but raises housing costs by imposing unnecessary requirements and delays, and restrictive rules that stifle diversity and limit consumer choice on the other.

This discussion demonstrates rather convincingly that Western Europe and North America have shared a remarkably similar set of experiences regarding shelter and service issues for the elderly. We have borrowed ideas from each other, we have learned from each other and as a consequence, our ever emerging responses have without question improved the quality of life for our collective elders and will no doubt continue to do so.

Chapter 2

Housing and Household Movement in Later Life: Developing the Range of Housing Options in the United Kingdom

Anthea Tinker

SUMMARY. In most developed countries housing policies are focusing on enabling elderly and very elderly people to remain in their own homes. Attention is also turning to people in the Third Age to see how their housing needs to be different from earlier stages of their lives but also as a preparation for old age. This paper presents evidence from the United Kingdom (UK) about choices and policies at different stages of middle and old age and on the developing range of housing options to meet these needs. *[Article copies available for a fee from The Haworth Document Delivery Service: 1-800-342-9678. E-mail address: getinfo@haworth.com]*

Anthea Tinker, PhD, is Professor of Social Gerontology, and Director, Age Concern Institute of Gerontology, King's College London, Cornwall House Annexe, Waterloo Road, London SE1 8TX, England.

Material from the General Household Survey made available through the Office of Population Censuses and Surveys and the Economic and Social Research Archive has been used by permission of the Controller of HMSO. The data was analyzed by the Gerontology Data Service at the Age Concern Institute of Gerontology, King's College London.

[Haworth co-indexing entry note]: "Housing and Household Movement in Later Life: Developing the Range of Housing Options in the United Kingdom." Tinker, Anthea. Co-published simultaneously in *Journal of Housing for the Elderly* (The Haworth Press, Inc.) Vol. 12, No. 1/2, 1997, pp. 9-17; and: *Shelter and Service Issues for Aging Populations: International Perspectives* (ed: Leon A. Pastalan) The Haworth Press, Inc., 1997, pp. 9-17. Single or multiple copies of this article are available for a fee from The Haworth Document Delivery Service [1-800-342-9678, 9:00 a.m. - 5:00 p.m. (EST). E-mail address: getinfo@haworth.com].

INTRODUCTION

A theme of policies in many developed countries is a commitment to enabling elderly people in their own homes. In practice this is where the majority do live. For example, in the Organization for Economic Cooperation and Development (OECD) countries, approximately 90% of elderly people, including a percentage who are frail, live in ordinary non-specialized accommodation. In the UK only approximately 5-6% of elderly people live in institutional care. In some other countries there has been more emphasis on institutional care in the past.

Recent research has demonstrated the neglect of housing in community care plans, both in the UK and elsewhere (Tinker, 1994). Nevertheless, the importance of home to elderly people, for practical and psychological reasons, is gaining a higher profile. For example, the OECD commissioned research on the role of housing for frail elderly people as part of their concern about policies for this group (Tinker, 1994).

The topics to be covered in this paper are:

- Demographic Constraints (trends and household movements)
- The Choices of Elderly People
- Policies for Frail and Elderly People
- Housing in the Third Age
- Some Issues

DEMOGRAPHIC CONSTRAINTS

In the United Kingdom the large growth in the proportion of the population who are elderly has already taken place. From now until the end of the century numbers and proportions will change little. After that the proportion of people aged 60-74 will increase but not as dramatically as those over the age of 75. The latter is largely a reflection of previous high fertility and improvements in late age mortality. It is also expected that those in their third age (usually defined as people aged 50-74) will increase. As Warnes has shown, there will be a substantial growth in this sector of the population from the late 1990s (Warnes, 1993). Between 1989-2020 "it is expected that there will be a 35% increase in the third age population, and a 28% increase in the female population. A recession will come after 2020, when the low 1970s and 1980s birth cohorts reach their third age" (Warnes, 1993, p. 28). It must of course be made clear that projections are based on a number of factors including the unpredictable fertility rates as well as assumptions about late age mortality.

It should also be noted that a growing proportion of elderly people live alone (Askham et al., 1992). In the UK in 1988, 32% of the over 60s lived alone, 49% with a spouse, 9% with a spouse and others and 10% with others (not a spouse). For those who are over the age of 75, many more live alone–50% and fewer with a spouse (34%). As with all demographic data there are marked differences between men and women (see Askham et al., 1992).

Elderly people in the UK are not a particularly mobile group. Whereas the 1981 census showed that 10% of the whole population moved in the previous year, only 5% of people over the age of 65 had moved. Most moves are of a short distance. Moves are usually of three types–to another tenure, to a retirement area or to be near relatives. It appears that there is a slight peak in migration at 65 and then a second peak in later old age. People who move are not typical. They tend to be more likely to be owner occupiers, married couples, those with relatively few dependent children and in good health (Warnes, 1993, p. 81).

THE CHOICES FOR ELDERLY PEOPLE

There are many different housing choices to make in old age. This section will discuss four of these:

- Type of Home
- Tenure
- Town or Country?
- To Stay or to Move?

Type of Home

The majority of elderly people in the UK live in houses. In 1988, 83% of households containing two adults, of whom one or both were aged 60 or over, lived in houses, 15% in a purpose built flat or maisonette and 2% in a converted flat, maisonette or rooms. What many old people seem to want is somewhere small and easy to manage. Table 1 shows that the choice of a house declines as people age and preference for both bungalows and flats increases.

Tenure

For all households in the UK the major change has been the rise in owner occupation. Whereas 44% of all households owned their own home

TABLE 1. Preferred type of accommodation (if considering a move) by age of head of household: Great Britain, 1988.

Preferred type of dwelling	30-44 years %	45-59 years %	60-69 years %	70-79 years %	80 years & over %
Detached *house*	56	32	12	6	3
Semi-detached *house*	9	8	6	4	3
Terraced *house*	3	2	2	3	2
House	4	2	2	2	2
Bungalow	23	47	63	58	52
Flat	3	5	11	21	22
Other	2	3	5	7	16
Total	100	99	101	101	100
Sample size	2,824	2,381	1,687	1,400	616

Source: OPCS General Household Survey, 1988

Source: Warnes (ed.) (1992) The Carnegie Inquiry into the Third Age

in 1959, that figure had risen to 64% in 1988. The proportion of the over-sixties owning their own home rose from 46% in 1979 to 57% in 1988. The greatest changes have been for the young elderly. At the same time, the proportion of elderly people living in local authority housing dropped from 37% in 1979 to 32% in 1988. Whether owner occupation will continue to hold such an attraction is difficult to forecast.

Town or Country?

The majority of elderly people in the UK live in an urban environment. Preference for country living appears to decline with age. The 1978 General Household Survey (GHS) asked people "whether, if they were considering moving somewhere else, they would prefer to live in the town or the country. Preference for the country declined consistently, being preferred by 59% of those aged 30-44 years, 56% of those aged 45-59, 51% of those aged 60-64 and only 38% of the over eighties" (Askham, 1992, p. 88).

To Stay or to Move?

As has been seen, older people are not a particularly mobile group. There are many well-known advantages of staying put. These include familiarity with the home, neighborhood links and the sense of continuity with the past that home gives. Research, as has already been indicated, shows that some people move unwillingly into sheltered housing. The same is true of residential care. On the other hand, homes may become too large, difficult to manage, heat and repair. They may also be too far from amenities such as shops and from sources of informal support such as relatives.

Table 2 shows that about three quarters of people in the third age and over 75 would prefer to remain in their present home if they had a free choice. This contrasts with only half of people under the age of 50. What is clear is the need for advice so that decisions are not taken in haste.

POLICIES FOR FRAIL ELDERLY PEOPLE

Although disability increases with age, there should be no assumption that older people necessarily need special housing. Appropriate housing is needed at all ages of life although the likelihood of suffering some form of mental or physical disability increases at a greater rate after the age of 75. As has been seen, most elderly people wish to remain in their own homes and attention is increasingly focusing on this. There are two major housing policies (moving to residential care is of course another option but is not within the scope of this paper as it is not housing):

- staying at home with a package of care, and
- moving to supported housing such as very sheltered housing.

TABLE 2. Whether people would choose to stay in their present home or move if they had a free choice by age, 1990.

Preference to move or stay	Under 50 years %	50-74 years %	75 years and over %
Stay here	54	71	79
Move elsewhere	44	26	20
Don't know/no answer	2	3	1
Total	100	100	100
Sample size	822	422	96

Source: British Social Attitudes Survey 1990-

Source: Warnes (ed.) (1992) The Carnegie Inquiry into the Third Age

Staying at Home with a Package of Care

If an elderly person is in need of help, this can be of different kinds. It may be that help is needed with personal and domestic tasks, with the home or there may be a problem in communicating with sources of help. The development in the UK has been the responsibility given to local authority social services departments to assess elderly people who are in need of services. This can be for residential services departments or domiciliary services. They have a statutory obligation to consult users and caregivers. In the overall design of services for the area they must consult health, housing, the voluntary sector and users and caregivers. For individuals who are assessed as needing care at home, a package of care must be designed.

It is not the purpose of this paper to go into details of the help for domiciliary and personal tasks but for help with the home and for communications, the input of housing is crucial. The poor state of housing of some elderly people, despite improvements in the 1980s, is still evident. Although the greatest improvement in conditions between 1981 and 1986 was in homes occupied by people aged 75 and over, this group was more likely than other groups to have homes which were unfit or lacking amenities (see Tinker, 1992). There is also need for elderly people to have help in their homes with minor problems such as wiring and insulation.

A range of grants are available from local authorities and these are, in the main, means tested. What many older people need, however, is help with getting grants and getting their homes improved and repaired. One of the most encouraging developments in the UK has been the development of agency services to help owner occupiers. Agency services can be provided by local authorities, housing associations, voluntary bodies and the private sector. They provide advice and practical assistance. Their help is usually technical and financial and can include assistance with raising money (through grants, loans, etc.) for the work, help with choice, organization and supervision of builders and checking that the work has been satisfactorily completed. Research has shown them to provide a good quality service and an expansion was recommended (Leather and Mackintosh, 1990).

The need to communicate with others both in an emergency and for social contact has been largely met by the development of alarms. The use of telephones, however, especially as a way of relatives and older people keeping in touch should not be ignored. The extent of telephone coverage in the UK is not as high as in some other developed countries. While 87% of the over 60s owned a telephone in 1988, only 80% of those aged 80 and over did (Askham et al., 1992). Butler (1989) has illustrated the potential for alarms for different purposes. In the UK the main use is for the first two categories, i.e., emergency calls and speech conversation and reassurance. The use of alarms for body monitoring is used for other groups but very little for older people. Nevertheless, it has great potential for frail elderly people. Electronic tagging has been used in a few cases in residential care homes but is controversial because of the ethical issues involved.

A Move to Supported Housing Such as Very Sheltered Housing

One of the most interesting recent developments in the UK has been the provision of very sheltered or extra care housing. This is sheltered housing with more provision or a greater level of care than ordinary sheltered housing, for example with provision of meals, extra wardens, domiciliary assistants or additional communal facilities. In 1985, 17% of local authorities and 11% of housing associations in England and Wales made this kind of provision and 24% of non-providing local authorities and 14% of non-providing housing associations were planning schemes. An evaluation showed that they were liked by staff, management and tenants (Tinker, 1989). They were found to be more expensive than staying at home options but very much cheaper than hospitals and slightly cheaper than local authority residential care. Turning existing, or parts of sheltered housing into very sheltered was suggested as a future option as well as new build.

HOUSING IN THE THIRD AGE

A study of housing in the Third Age was recently undertaken for the Carnegie Inquiry into the Third Age (Warnes, ed., 1992). Striking overall features were the improvement in housing standards as well as the rise in owner occupation. However, great diversity was found. There was a strong relationship with income, occupational group, ethnic group and region. Concern was expressed about low income groups who, if they are owner occupiers, may not be able to repair their homes. The decline in public sector building of small specially designed housing was also a matter of concern. In addition "A small number of people in the third age, particularly those who experience severe income decline following bereavement or divorce, may default on mortgage interest payments, and be contributing to the worrying rise in house possessions and even homelessness" (Warnes, ed., 1992, p. xi).

SOME ISSUES

Against the background of a developing range of housing options there are a number of issues which arise. These are to do with the housing itself, affordability, support services, the need for advice and some are to do with particular groups.

On housing there is concern that there is enough appropriate housing. For older people who wish to move there is a lack of small housing despite a switch from the provision of 3 bedroom family houses to smaller accommodation. While many elderly people could be satisfactorily housed in ordinary non-specialized housing, the drop in the building of sheltered, including very sheltered, housing must be looked at in the context of an increasing number and proportion of very elderly people. A recent study by the Department of the Environment of Housing Needs and Provision gives estimates of what might be needed and who is thought to be suitable for what form of housing (McCafferty, 1994). It found that two out of three elderly households had no assessed need for any form of subsidized specialized housing or other housing without care support. Of those households that did have a need for provision, seven out of ten wished to remain at home and could be enabled to do so with repairs and adaptations to their homes and/or domiciliary support. On a national scale there was evidence of over-provision of traditional or ordinary sheltered housing with warden support and communal facilities and an under-provision of very sheltered housing with extra-care support. A strong case can also be made for an extension of agency schemes to help elderly owner occupiers.

Affordability, especially for those who rent, is of prime importance for older people whose incomes are likely to decline in old age. In the UK, local authority rents are rising and there is concern that the new funding arrangements for housing associations will force rents up beyond the reach of older people.

Support services, such as home care, are essential for frail elderly people. There is concern that the social workers who will carry out the assessments will not be sufficiently knowledgeable or skilled to carry it out. There is also a fear that the services will not be extensive enough to cover all the potential demand.

The need for advice, including whether people should move or not, is crucial. A great deal of unhappiness could be prevented if elderly people and their caregivers could discuss the options in advance of a crisis.

The needs of particular groups are beyond the scope of this paper but the needs of older women, homeless elderly people and those from black and ethnic minority groups must be mentioned.

REFERENCES

Askham, J. (1992) 'Attitudes of people in the third age' in Warnes (ed.), pp. 84-90.

Askham, J., Barry, C., Grundy, E., Hancock, R. and Tinker, A. (1992) *Life After Sixty*, Age Concern Institute of Gerontology, King's College London.

Butler, A. (1989) 'The Growth and development of alarm systems in sheltered housing' in Fisk, J. (ed.), *Alarm Systems and Elderly People*, The Planning Exchange, Glasgow, Scotland, pp. 110-128.

Leather, P. and Mackintosh, S. (1990) *Monitoring Assisted Agency Services. Part 1: Home Improvement Agencies—An Evaluation of Performance*, HMSO, London.

McCafferty, P. (1994) *Living Independently: A Study of the Housing Needs of Elderly and Disabled People*, HMSO, London.

Tinker, A. (1989) *An Evaluation of Very Sheltered Housing*, HMSO, London.

Tinker, A. (1992) *Elderly People in Modern Society*, Longman, London.

Tinker, A. (1994) 'The role of housing policies in the care of elderly people' in Hennessy, P. (ed.), *Caring for Frail Elderly People: New Directions in Care*, OECD, Paris, pp. 57-82.

Warnes, T. (ed.) (1992) *Homes and Travel: Local Life in the Third Age*, Carnegie UK Trust, Fife, Scotland.

Warnes, A.W. (1993) *The Demography of Ageing in the United Kingdom of Great Britain and Northern Ireland*, National Institute on Aging, Malta.

Chapter 3

Housing Older Canadians:
Current Patterns, Preferences and Policies

Andrew Wister
Gloria Gutman

SUMMARY. Reflecting a world-wide trend toward avoidance of institutionalization and the fostering of aging in place in the community, a range of housing alternatives has been developed for older persons in Canada. This paper examines: (1) current patterns of housing and living arrangements of older Canadians; (2) philosophies that have dominated policy and production of housing for seniors for the last 30 years; and (3) seniors' preferences and utilization rates of various options. Data sources include the 1991 census and two cross-Canada studies, one urban and one rural, in which seniors were asked about their housing and related support service needs, usage patterns and preferences. The paper concludes with a discussion of emerging trends blending shelter and services and of policy gaps that need to be addressed in meeting the future housing needs of older Canadians. *[Article copies available for a fee from The Haworth Document Delivery Service: 1-800-342-9678. E-mail address: getinfo@ haworth.com]*

Andrew Wister, PhD, and Gloria Gutman, PhD, are affiliated with the Gerontology Research Centre, Simon Fraser University at Harbour Centre, 2800-515 West Hastings Street, Vancouver, British Columbia, Canada, V6B 5K3.

An earlier version of this paper was presented as part of a roundtable discussion on "Current Trends in Housing and Housing Policy" held at the 15th World Congress of Gerontology, Budapest, Hungary, July 4-9, 1993.

[Haworth co-indexing entry note]: "Housing Older Canadians: Current Patterns, Preferences and Policies." Wister, Andrew, and Gloria Gutman. Co-published simultaneously in *Journal of Housing for the Elderly* (The Haworth Press, Inc.) Vol. 12, No. 1/2, 1997, pp. 19-35; and: *Shelter and Service Issues for Aging Populations: International Perspectives* (ed: Leon A. Pastalan) The Haworth Press, Inc., 1997, pp. 19-35. Single or multiple copies of this article are available for a fee from The Haworth Document Delivery Service [1-800-342-9678, 9:00 a.m. - 5:00 p.m. (EST). E-mail address: getinfo@haworth.com].

INTRODUCTION

This paper begins with an overview of the housing and living arrangements of older persons living in Canada today. The second part of the paper reviews three philosophic approaches that have dominated policy and production of housing for seniors in Canada over the last 30 years:

- Construction of institutions and purpose built housing.
- Promotion of housing alternatives and maximization of housing choice.
- Aging in place.

The third and final part of the paper focuses on current approaches which are distinguished from their predecessors by a deliberate attempt to blend shelter and services so as to enable the semi-independent elderly to remain longer in the community.

PART I:
AN OVERVIEW OF HOUSING AND LIVING ARRANGEMENTS OF OLDER CANADIANS

In 1991, when the most recent Canadian census was conducted, persons aged 65 and over numbered 3,170,000 and constituted 11.6% of the population. Among Canadians aged 65 and over, 1,839,540 or 58.0% were women.

Age and Gender Differences in Living Arrangements

As shown in Table 1, the vast majority of older persons, both male and female, live in private households. In 1991, only 6.1% of males aged 65 and over and 10.3% of females were residents of "collective dwellings," defined by Statistics Canada as including: special care homes for the elderly and chronically ill, hospitals, religious institutions, hotels, motels, tourist homes, and other collective households such as jails, military camps, and work camps.

Within the category of private households, there are some major differences in the pattern of living arrangements between males and females, as well as between women under and over age 75. For example, the majority (75.8%) of men live in families with a spouse and/or never-married children. Even among men aged 75 and over, two-thirds (66.7%) live in such family settings. Among women, the proportion living in family arrange-

TABLE 1. The Elderly Population by Living Arrangement, Age and Sex: Canada, 1991

Living Arrangement	Total Pop. Aged 65 +		Ages 65-74		Ages 75 +	
	Male	Female	Male	Female	Male	Female
Private Households:						
Family Households	75.8%	50.0%	80.8%	62.0%	66.7%	34.2%
With Relatives	1.7%	3.9%	1.5%	3.3%	2.1%	4.8%
With Non-Relatives	2.2%	1.6%	2.2%	1.7%	2.0%	1.5%
Alone	14.3%	34.2%	12.4%	29.7%	17.5%	40.0%
Collective Dwellings	5.7%	9.9%	2.6%	2.9%	11.3%	19.2%

Source: Statistics Canada. 1991 Census. *Families: Number, Type and Structure.* Catalogue 93-312, Table 8, July, 1992; Statistics Canada. 1991 Census. *Dwellings and Households.* Catalogue 93-311, Table 2, July, 1992.

ments decreases dramatically with age–from 62.0% in the age group 65-74 to 34.2% among women 75+. There is a concomitant increase in the proportion living in non-family households, either alone in private households (29.7% of women aged 65-74; 40.0% of women aged 75+) or as residents of "collective dwellings" (2.9% of women aged 65-74; 19.2% of women aged 75+).

The large proportion of older women living alone is a relatively new phenomenon; between 1961 and 1991, the proportion of Canadian women aged 65 and over living alone more than doubled (from 16% to 34.2%).

Type and Size of Dwellings Occupied by Older Canadians

Table 2 shows that even in the 75 and over age group, most males (61.4%) live in a single family detached house. While such dwellings are also the most common housing form occupied by women (45.7% in the age group 65-74 and 39.5% among women 75+), substantially more

TABLE 2. Private Households of Elderly Population by Structural Type, Age and Sex of Primary Maintainer*

Structural Type	Total pop. 65 +		Ages 65-74		Ages 75 +	
	Male	Female	Male	Female	Male	Female
Single - detached home	66.1%	42.7%	68.4%	45.7%	61.4%	39.5%
Apt. - 5 or more storeys	10.3%	21.3%	8.7%	18.2%	13.7%	24.7%
Movable dwelling	1.8%	1.2%	1.8%	1.4%	1.7%	0.9%
Other**	21.8%	34.8%	21.2%	34.7%	23.2%	34.9%

* 20% sample data

** Includes "semi-detached home," "row house," "other single house attached," "apartment in a detached duplex," and "apartment in a building fewer than 5 storeys."

Source: Statistics Canada. 1991 Census. *Housing Costs and Other Characteristics of Canadian Households.* Catalogue 93-330, Table 2, May, 1993.

women than men live in apartments and other forms of multi-unit housing. Table 3 shows that the dwellings occupied by older females are generally smaller than those occupied by males.

Age and Gender Differences in Housing Tenure

Chevan (1987) reported that in the United States, between 1940 and 1980, the proportion of persons aged 65 and over who owned their own home increased from 46% to about 63%. Over the same time period, the trend was the same in Canada. Currently, 66.1% of private household maintainers aged 65 and over occupy self-owned dwellings.

Table 4 shows private households by tenure and the age and gender of the primary maintainer. As can be seen, among males even in the 75+ age group, a majority (71.4%) own their own home. Home ownership is less common among female maintainers.

While most of the homes owned by elderly persons in Canada are single family detached dwellings, the number of seniors purchasing condominiums is increasing, particularly in some parts of the country. In 1991, 5.3% of Canadian seniors owned condominiums, up from 1.8% in

TABLE 3. Private Households of Elderly Population by Size of Dwelling and Age and Sex of Primary Maintainer: Canada, 1991

	average no. of bedrooms		average no. rooms per dwelling		average no. persons per household		average no. persons per room	
Age	Male	Female	Male	Female	Male	Female	Male	Female
65-74	2.7	2.2	6.0	5.1	2.1	1.4	.4	.3
75 +	2.4	1.9	5.5	4.7	1.9	1.3	.3	.3

Source: Statistics Canada. 1991 Census. *Housing Costs and Other Characteristics of Canadian Households.* Catalogue 93-330, Table 2, May, 1993.

TABLE 4. Private Households of Elderly Population by Tenure, Age and Sex of Primary Maintainer: Canada, 1991*

Tenure	Total pop. 65 +		65-74		75 +	
	Male	Female	Male	Female	Male	Female
Owned						
Condo	5.2	5.4	4.9	6.0	5.7	4.7
Non-Condo	71.3	46.3	74.1	49.9	65.7	42.3
Rented	23.5	48.3	21.0	44.0	28.7	53.0

*   20% sample data

Source: Statistics Canada. 1991 Census. *Housing Costs and Other Characteristics of Canadian Households.* Catalogue 93-330, Table 2, May, 1993.

1981. The proportion owning condominiums in the west coast province of British Columbia was 13% in 1991, up from 8.3% in 1981.

Living Alone

As noted above, over the last 30 years there has been a dramatic increase in the proportion of Canadian seniors, particularly women, living alone in private households. In fact, the number of people of all ages living alone has more than doubled since 1961. Statistics Canada (1993) attributes this trend in part to the overall aging of the population, in part to an increase in marriage breakups and, in the upper age groups, to the gender difference in mortality rates. (Currently in Canada, life expectancy at birth is 79.89 for females compared with 72.95 for males.)

Priest (1985, 1988) notes that, in addition to the dramatic increase in the proportion of Canadian seniors living alone in private households, the proportion living in institutions has increased. Conversely, over the same 30-year period, we have witnessed a significant decrease, particularly among those aged 75 and over, in the proportion of older adults living in the homes of their children. There are a number of factors contributing to these trends, including increased income (Priest, 1985, 1988), lower fertility, greater availability of purpose-built seniors housing, greater availability of institutional beds, as well as, and perhaps most importantly, seniors' expressed desire to remain independent for as long as possible (Kobrin, 1976; Michael, Fuchs & Scott, 1980; Wister, 1989).

For many Canadian seniors, remaining independent is synonymous with living separate from their children. This does not mean that they are divorced from or abandoned by their children. Rather, it reflects a widely held preference for what has been called "intimacy at a distance" (Rosenmayr & Kockeis, 1963). However, at a personal level, we believe that this preference for independence should be recognized as an expression of and a direct result of older persons', and especially older women's, empowerment. Evidence for this interpretation is provided in a set of studies conducted by Dr. Veronica Doyle. In these studies (Doyle & Rafferty, 1991), a group of 12 older women who live alone designed and conducted interviews with 175 other older women living alone and discovered that a key theme underlying their choice of living arrangement was a belief that "it's my turn now." That is, after a lifetime of looking after others, these women had actively chosen to live alone, and in some cases at risk, in order to be able "to do what they want to do when they want to do it."

The remainder of this paper discusses the evolution of Canada's housing policies and programs for older persons and where we see them heading.

PART II:
PHILOSOPHIES AND APPROACHES
TO HOUSING OLDER CANADIANS, 1960-1990

Haldemann and Wister (1993) identify three distinct approaches to dealing with shelter and care of the aged in Canada over the last 30 years, each of which has developed in succession by building on the foundation of the preceding models but shifting the relative importance of the resources attributed to each.

Approach 1: Construction of Institutions and Purpose-Built Seniors' Housing

The first approach, which was observed in the 1960s and 1970s, consisted of the construction of institutions (variously called nursing homes, homes for the aged, or chronic care homes) as well as, simultaneously, the construction of purpose-built housing for older persons.

As Haldemann and Wister note:

> ... After the traditional asylum for the poor, the nursing home was offered by the new welfare state to the elderly as an alternative for people who could not stay at home for a wide variety of reasons (health, income, social isolation, etc.) ... With the rising demand for nursing homes during the 1970s and the concomitant rise in costs, access to this kind of shelter was restricted to people with serious health problems. (p. 31)

The housing constructed during this period, on the other hand, was targeted from the outset at well-elderly with income problems. Under Section 53.1 of the National Housing Act, non-profit groups from across the country received financial assistance in the form of low interest mortgages from the Canada Mortgage and Housing Corporation (CMHC) to build housing for low-income seniors. The stipulation was that seniors would not be required to pay more than 30% of their income for rent and that the buildings would offer shelter only. As Appleyard (1994) has pointed out, sponsoring groups were told not to worry about the seniors who, virtually from the day these buildings opened, would get sick and/or require some degree of assistance with activities of daily living. The assumption was that these individuals would willingly move out when they were no longer fully independent. While there was some recognition that relocation could have a negative impact on older persons, no one was thinking much about the long-term. We knew little about transition rates; the underlying belief was that people would move into seniors' housing in good health and, after a few years, die suddenly in their suite or shortly after admission to an acute hospital or, suffer a catastrophic illness such as a stroke or heart attack which, if they survived, would necessitate a move to a nursing home. We didn't expect them to linger on for 10 or even 20 years in seniors' housing.

During the late 1970s and throughout the 1980s, especially in the Canadian provinces of British Columbia, Manitoba, and Ontario, there was growing interest and development of publicly funded home care (Meals on Wheels, homemakers, adult day care). The predictable outcome of this development, which was accompanied by a slow down or, in some jurisdictions, a moratorium on the construction of publicly funded institutional beds, was that the average age of the nursing home population increased considerably (e.g., in B.C. the average age in nursing homes in 1978-79 was 75; currently it is 85). Residents are also much more frail at the time of admission than in 1978-79. (We will discuss the implications of this for housing later.)

Approach 2: Housing Alternatives and Maximization of Choice

Haldemann and Wister (1993) note that in the late 1970s, recognition of the heterogeneity of the older population, accentuated by growing numbers of people leaving the labour force at younger ages and by the very old surviving longer, made it more difficult to promote a single model of shelter as the ideal for all or even a majority of seniors. Throughout the 1980s the key words were "choices" and "alternatives."

CMHC held a series of conferences and developed publications (e.g., CMHC, 1988a, 1988b, 1989) designed to make seniors and developers aware of the range of housing alternatives potentially available. This range included "sheltered housing," "congregate housing," "granny flats" (called "garden suites" by CMHC), "homesharing" and financial vehicles such as reverse annuity mortgages and life tenancies. However, both the market place and research studies have shown that many of these options appeal to only a small percentage of seniors.

For example, a 1989 survey was conducted in three rural areas in Canada (Gutman & Hodge, 1990) in which the following 14 options were inquired about:

For Both Owners and Renters

> Purchasing a unit in *special retirement housing* which, respondents were told, was "a housing development especially built for seniors, not a nursing home."
>
> Moving into *sheltered housing* which was described as "a type of seniors housing that consists of self-contained apartments or small one-storey homes that are clustered in projects of 20 to 50 units. A

key feature is that each unit is linked to the project manager by an alarm system."

Moving into *congregate housing*, which respondents were told "differs from sheltered housing primarily in terms of the number of services provided. Residents have their own private apartments which usually include a kitchen so that they can prepare light meals, but the main meals are eaten in a communal dining room. Housekeeping and personal care services are also usually included as a part of the accommodation package."

Hiring a *live-in housekeeper.*

Sharing a housekeeper in an *Abbeyfield House* arrangement, described to respondents as follows: "some people (usually 7 to 10) have moved into a large house called an *Abbeyfield House*, where they have their own private room and share one or more meals a day and the services of a housekeeper in a family atmosphere. The house is acquired and operated by a non-profit society but the residents share in the operation of the house.

Moving into a *garden suite* which, after telling respondents was otherwise known as "a granny flat," was described as a small self-contained house that is placed on the same lot as the home of a family member. It is designed for older people, they were told, "who want to live close to their children while maintaining their independence and privacy. Most suites have one bedroom, a living room, a kitchen, a bathroom, as well as storage and laundry facilities. The suites are not intended as permanent additions to the lots. They are usually factory-built and can be quickly erected and easily moved when no longer needed."

Purchasing a *mobile home* in a planned retirement community.

Purchasing shares in *cooperative housing*. Here respondents were told "members of a co-op share in both the ownership and the management of the complex they live in. After initially buying shares, they make monthly payments which cover part of the building's mortgage, interest, and operating costs. This gives them the right to occupy a specific unit. When they leave, their shares are redeemed by the co-op."

For Owners Only

> *Buying a smaller single family detached house.*

> Entering into a *homesharing arrangement* described as "an arrangement where two or more *unrelated* people live together in a dwelling unit. Each has a private space while sharing common areas such as bathroom, kitchen, living and dining room. In most cases one person owns the home and the other pays rent or provides some services to the homeowner such as cooking, housekeeping or gardening in exchange for free or reduced rent."

> Adapting their existing home to *put in a private suite* that can be rented out.

> Taking out a *Reverse Annuity Mortgage,* described as "a plan that allows seniors to have extra income by using their equity–or the value–they've built up in their home. Under this plan, an older homeowner would take out a mortgage on his or her home and the plan guarantees the home owner a monthly income for a fixed period of time (usually 10-15 years) or, in some plans, for life. The mortgage and interest don't have to be repaid until the fixed term expires or the owner dies or the home is sold."

> Entering into a *Life-Tenancy Arrangement,* explained to respondents as follows: "Another thing some people do is sell some of the equity in their home while retaining occupancy rights. There are two basic ways people can do this. They can sell their home to an investor, who immediately leases it back to the seller for life. The seller becomes a renter in the home he or she has just sold. This is called *sale-lease-back.* The other way of doing it is called a *life hold estate.* In this case you again sell your home to an investor but the title to the property doesn't transfer until the owner dies."

> Deferring their property taxes until they die or the property is sold, at which time the taxes plus interest are due.

As shown in Table 5, which presents the combined "yes" and "maybe, I'll consider" responses to these options, the most popular in all three regions and among both owners and renters were *sheltered housing* and *congregate housing.* From one-third to one-half of all groups indicated that they would consider these two housing forms. One-third to one-half of

TABLE 5. Housing Option Preferences of Rural Seniors, by Tenure Type and Region

	% "yes" and "maybe" would consider:					
	Owners			Renters		
Housing Option:	CKRD	WPC	KC	CKRD*	WPC	KC
	(n = 175)	(n = 102)	(n = 39)	(n = 13)	(n = 72)	(n = 19)
Owners and Renters						
Sheltered housing	54.9	52.0	38.5	--	30.6	47.4
Congregate housing	47.4	45.1	35.9	--	34.7	42.1
Retirement housing	48.6	52.0	33.3	--	13.9	26.3
Garden suite	24.0	34.3	28.2	--	16.7	21.1
Mobile home	30.3	28.4	12.8	--	11.1	15.8
Live-in housekeeper	15.4	26.5	35.9	--	9.7	15.8
Abbeyfield House	11.4	18.6	20.5	--	12.5	10.5
Co-op housing	13.1	18.6	15.4	--	4.2	10.5
Owners Only						
Homesharing	24.6	20.6	20.5			
Buying smaller house	24.6	21.6	15.4			
Reverse annuity mortgage	13.1	12.7	17.9		N/A	
Life tenancy arrangement	9.1	5.9	20.5			
Adding a suite	9.7	10.8	5.6			
Deferring property taxes	10.3	3.9	10.3			

*Question not asked.

Source: Gutman and Hodge (1990)

the owners in all three regions would also consider *purchasing a unit in a special retirement housing.*

The next most popular group of options for owners were, in order of the proportion who would consider them: moving into a garden suite, purchasing a smaller home, purchasing a mobile home, homesharing, and hiring a live-in housekeeper. For all these options, there was at least one owner group in which one-quarter to one-third said they would consider it.

Considerably less popular was the idea of purchasing shares in co-op housing, moving into an Abbeyfield House, taking out a reverse annuity mortgage, adding a revenue suite, entering into a life-tenancy arrangement and deferring property taxes. In all groups, fewer than 21% of owners said they would consider these options.

In interpreting these data, it should be noted that there were generally more "maybe" than "yes, I would seriously consider" responses to these options. The market for them, in other words, is probably less than the findings suggest.

In support of this argument it should be noted that 10.3% of the respondents from one rural region (CKRD) said "yes" or "maybe" they would consider deferring their property taxes. Data from the 1988 Household Income, Facilities and Equipment Survey (Statistics Canada, 1988) indicated however, that among seniors in that province who were eligible to take advantage of The Land Tax Deferment Program, only 1.9% actually did so!

In summary, the data from the rural seniors study and a study conducted with urban seniors (Gutman, Milstein & Doyle, 1987) suggest that many of these housing options appeal to only a small proportion of the seniors' population. It is important that in fostering these options, governments do not lose sight of the need to support the construction of low cost rental accommodation. Using as the criterion of excessive housing burden the expenditure of more than 30% of income for shelter, it must be recognized that among seniors, affordability is much more a renters' than an owners' problem (Gutman, 1990; Struyk, 1977). In Canada, it is also both an urban problem, since the bulk of seniors live in urban centres, and a women's problem since there are more older women than older men who fall in low income categories (Gutman, in press).

Approach 3: Aging in Place

As Haldemann and Wister note, aging in place, the watchword of the '80s, implies adequate housing. Recognizing that in some cases the homes seniors were being asked to stay in were not adequate, during the 1980s the federal government, through CMHC, developed or extended several programs that made funds available to seniors and/or disabled persons to make structural repairs to their dwellings (e.g., fix broken stairs or a leaky roof; add ramps, grab bars, a stair lift or make other adaptations that compensate for physical disabilities). CMHC also fostered the development of a self-help tool (Maltais, Trickey & Robitaille, 1989) for identifying ways in which the home environment did not fit the users' needs and might be modified.

During the 1980s, a number of provinces instituted shelter allowance programs for elderly renters in the belief that this would enable these individuals to move into units that would better meet their needs and/or enable them to stay put in a rising rental market that otherwise would exceed their ability to pay. The view was that seniors had an income rather than a housing problem and so, if they had a bit more money, the housing problem would be resolved.

Despite the studies referred to above that have suggested minimal interest in equity liquidation, in the late 1980s and early 1990s, the CMHC has promoted reverse annuity mortgages and other financial vehicles that would enable seniors to use the equity in their homes to finance the cost of repairs, upgrading, taxes, etc.

One sector that was largely ignored were projects built under "shelter-only" policies. With respect to these, it is important to note that many of the social housing units that were built for seniors in the 1960s and 1970s were bachelor (studio) units. At the time that these were constructed, the thinking was that seniors require only basic shelter. It is now clear that more is needed. As the occupants of these units have aged in place, their needs have changed. The characteristics of new tenants have also changed. Some years ago, Lawton, Greenbaum and Liebowitz (1980) noted that replacement tenants tended to be more like what the original tenants had become than what they were like when they first entered a project (i.e., replacement tenants were more frail at entry than the original tenants had been). As Appleyard (1994) notes, government cutbacks in construction of nursing home beds have exacerbated the problem. Today, housing projects are both retaining more frail tenants than they might otherwise do if nursing home beds were more readily available and, they are admitting tenants in more frail condition because these individuals have nowhere else to go. Unfortunately, many projects are not equipped to meet the changed characteristics of the tenant population. For example, many do not have the space and/or the wiring in place to enable a kitchen and communal dining room to be added. Where suites have been taken out of service and converted to other uses (e.g., as a dining room or doctor's office), in some jurisdictions projects have run into trouble with CMHC for having violated the terms under which they originally received mortgage financing.

> One example of the ensuing problems concerns . . . residents . . . who were hospitalized for malnutrition in spite of the availability of Meals on Wheels. Unable to stand by and do nothing, we converted two bachelor suites to a kitchen and a dining room and offered our residents a full course dinner once a day. This was probably the single best thing we ever did. However, it triggered a ten year fight with CMHC. They were concerned that the suites were not being used for shelter and that the kitchen, being small, was losing money. (Appleyard, 1994)

PART III:
BLENDING SHELTER AND SERVICES

Currently, a fourth approach is emerging in Canada that recognizes the need to interface shelter and care in more flexible arrangements than heretofore has been the case.

When dealing with seniors, it is unrealistic to think that a project can offer only shelter. Whether equipped for it or not, staff of shelter-only projects are called upon to assist elderly tenants in a variety of ways (Appleyard, 1994). Publically-funded home care in Canada has tended to be tied to the person rather than the project, meaning that persons in shelter-only projects are eligible to receive Meals on Wheels, homemaker services, etc. But, it has become apparent that this is not always the most effective and efficient use of resources. Alternative arrangements, such as allowing shelter-only projects to offer services as part of the rent, may be a better way of meeting changing tenants' needs.

Small group homes for persons with dementia, with generic staffing such as are common in Sweden, are another model currently being explored (Gallagher, 1993; Malmberg & Zarit, 1993). Some of the interface models will require the dismantling and blending of traditional boundaries and barriers between government ministries of health, housing, and social services. Other models, such as those involving generic staffing, will require changes of attitude and policy on the part of labour unions. Issues of licensing and inspection of the new breed of projects which fall between housing and institutions will also need to be addressed.

It would also be useful if we could develop a universally agreed upon and understood nomenclature for the various types of projects that fall in the mid-range of the shelter-care continuum. Is congregate housing the same thing as congregate care? Are sheltered housing and congregate housing terms that can be used synonymously? Is a small group home only a small group home if it is free-standing or, does the term include, as it sometimes seems to, a cluster of units within a multi-unit project?

CONCLUSION

In this paper, the evolution of housing policy in Canada has been described in terms of four philosophies or approaches, each of which has developed out of its predecessor. However, Canada has not had a clearly articulated housing policy that responds to the changing needs of older adults. The largest share of the housing program dollar goes to subsidized rents and home ownership grants. In fact, one trend in all policy in Canada is a shift from universal coverage to specificity in coverage (e.g., family allowance). Current housing policy appears to be moving away from the development and financial support of a range of housing options. Rather, specific areas are being investigated that will cost the federal and provincial governments less money. Concurrently, the private sector is being enticed to move into this field. Examples include a recent CMHC proposal (CMHC, 1992) that guarantees that private investors will suffer no losses if the market value of a property drops over the course of a "balloon payment mortgage." Although current preferences for such reverse annuities are low, they are being strongly promoted by housing officials, partly because they save the government money. Homesharing is an example of a previously supported program that is being phased out (most recently in Ontario) and left to the private sector. Equity co-ops, changing zoning to allow accessory apartments, and various forms of sheltered housing are receiving a fair amount of attention. Regarding equity co-ops, these are generally left up to groups to develop on their own unless they have a private or community organization assisting them. This raises the shelter-service interface issue and the need for intersectoral cooperation. Home care services also play a role in keeping people at home in the community, but we lack the research evidence that details their cost effectiveness.

What is clear is that we are moving into a period where specific groups need to be targeted in housing policy and research. All of the available data strongly suggest that older women living alone are severely at risk of poverty. We also can connect poverty with poor health. The need for enriched or sheltered housing continues to grow because more physically and cognitively disabled people are remaining out of institutions.

One of the problems that we are facing in attempting to ensure adequate housing for an aging population is the lack of coordination of services and shelter in a way that responds to a continuum of change in the individual. This is compounded by the inability of many people to anticipate, accept and respond to change in function. Thus, we need to recognize that there are limits to the efficacy of an aging in place philosophy. There is a growing problem of people who remain in place too long because there are few sheltered housing options and/or they fear institutions and the toll that this takes on family caregivers, many of whom themselves may be old and frail.

As we look towards the next century and attempt to delineate the principle housing and support issues and concerns for an aging population, it becomes apparent that future cohorts will likely be significantly different than their predecessors in their housing preferences, characteristics, and needs. Today's middle-aged Canadians have experienced higher rates of mobility and may therefore express lower levels of attachment to home in their later years. Demands for greater numbers of options and flexibility in housing may also be articulated by the baby-boom cohort. The sheer size of the older cohorts of the second and third decade of the next century may force greater attention onto housing problems of older adults. One thing is certain, however, for some time to come issues of poverty associated with earlier life stages (e.g., being a single-parent mother) will continue to drive demand for publically-funded housing for seniors and should be fundamental to our housing formulae of the future.

REFERENCES

Appleyard, R. (1994). Difficulties in providing support services in buildings constructed under shelter-only policies. In G. Gutman & A. Wister (Eds.), *Progressive Accommodation for Seniors: Interfacing Shelter and Care.* Vancouver: The Gerontology Research Centre, Simon Fraser University.

Canada Mortgage and Housing Corporation (CMHC) (1988a). *Housing Choices for Older Canadians.* Ottawa: The Corporation (Document NHA 6009).

Canada Mortgage and Housing Corporation (CMHC) (1988b). *Housing for Older Canadians: New Financial and Tenure Options.* Ottawa: The Corporation (Document NHA 6102).

Canada Mortgage and Housing Corporation (CMHC) (1989). *Conference Proceedings Options: Housing for Older Canadians.* Ottawa: The Corporation (Document NHA 6160).

Canada Mortgage and Housing Corporation (CMHC) (1992). *Consultation on Innovative Uses of Public Mortgage Loan Insurance.* Ottawa: The Corporation (Document NHA 6604-05).

Chevan, A. (1987). Homeownership in the older population: 1940-1980. *Research on Aging,* 9(2), 226-255.

Doyle, V. & Rafferty, P. (1991). The choice of older women to live alone: Action research by older women. Paper presented at the Annual Meeting of the Canadian Association on Gerontology, Toronto, October 24-27.

Gallagher, E. (1993). Group Homes: The Swedish model of care for persons with dementia of the Alzheimer's type. In G. Gutman & A. Wister (Eds.), *Progressive Accommodation for Seniors: Interfacing Shelter and Care.* Vancouver: The Gerontology Research Centre, Simon Fraser University.

Gutman, G.M. (1990). Seniors housing in B.C. Keynote address presented at the conference Choices Today, Options Tomorrow: Seniors' Housing for the 90's sponsored by the Canada Mortgage and Housing Corporation and the B.C. Housing Management Commission, Vancouver, June 25-27.

Gutman, G.M. (in press). Living arrangements, housing characteristics and poverty among Canada's older women. In J. Watzke, A. Wister & G. Gutman (Eds.), *Conference Proceedings "Older Women and Housing–Challenges and Choices."* Vancouver: The Gerontology Research Centre, Simon Fraser University.

Gutman, G.M. & Hodge, G. (1990). *Housing and Support Service Needs and Preferences of Rural Seniors from Three Regions in Canada.* Ottawa: Canada Mortgage and Housing Corporation.

Gutman, G.M., Milstein, S.L. & Doyle, V. (1987). *Attitudes of Seniors to Special Retirement Housing, Life Tenancy Arrangements and Other Housing Options.* Ottawa: Canada Mortgage and Housing Corporation.

Haldemann, V. & Wister, A. (1993). Environment and aging. *Journal of Canadian Studies,* 28(1), 30-43.

Kobrin, F. (1976). The fall in household size and the rise of the primary individual in the United States. *Demography,* 13(1), 127-138.

Lawton, M.P., Greenbaum, M. & Liebowitz, B. (1980). The lifespan of housing environments for the aging. *The Gerontologist,* 20(1), 56-64.

Malmberg, B. & Zarit, S.H. (1993). Group homes for people with dementia: A Swedish example. *The Gerontologist,* 33(5), 682-686.

Maltais, D., Trickey, F. & Robitaille, Y. (1989). *Maintaining Seniors Independence: A Guide to Home Adaptations.* Ottawa: Canada Mortgage and Housing Corporation.

Michael, R.T., Fuchs, V.R. & Scott, R. (1980). Changes in the propensity to live alone: Evidence from consecutive cross-sectional surveys. *Demography,* 17(1), 39-52.

Priest, G.E. (1985). *Living Arrangements of Canada's Elderly: Changing Demographic and Economic Factors.* Vancouver: The Gerontology Research Centre, Simon Fraser University. (Occasional Papers Series 85-1).

Priest, G.E. (1988). Living arrangements of Canada's older elderly. In G.M. Gutman & N.K. Blackie (Eds.), *Housing the Very Old.* Vancouver: The Gerontology Research Centre, Simon Fraser University.

Rosenmayr, L. & Kockeis, E. (1963). Propositions for a sociological theory of aging and the family. *International Social Science Journal,* 15, 410-426.

Statistics Canada (1988). *Survey of Household Income, Facilities and Equipment, 1988.*

Statistics Canada (1993). Solitaire, anyone? *Focus for the Future,* 6(3), 2.

Struyk, R.J. (1977). The housing expense burden of households headed by the elderly. *The Gerontologist,* 17, 447-452.

Wister, A.V. (1989). Privacy, independence and separateness in living arrangement selection among the elderly: Research and implications for housing policy. *Environments,* 20(2), 26-35.

Chapter 4

A Comparative Analysis
of Barrier-Free Housing:
Policies for Elderly People
in the United States and Canada

Peter A. Dunn

SUMMARY. This paper identifies policy issues in creating barrier-free housing for elderly people with disabilities in the United States and Canada. A range of policy options are described including: government housing construction; housing vouchers and certificates; community service programs; grants, loans and reimbursements; building codes and regulations; and human rights legislation. The strengths and weaknesses of these policy approaches are contrasted. The present emphasis in the United States is on individual housing rights compared with a more social welfare approach in Canada. Finally, one possible comprehensive model is described and practical next steps are outlined for making the housing environment more responsive to the needs of elderly people with disabilities. *[Article copies available for a fee from The Haworth Document Delivery Service: 1-800-342-9678. E-mail address: getinfo@haworth.com]*

Peter A. Dunn, PhD, is Associate Professor, Faculty of Social Work, Wilfrid Laurier University, Waterloo, Ontario, Canada N2L 3C5.

[Haworth co-indexing entry note]: "A Comparative Analysis of Barrier-Free Housing: Policies for Elderly People in the United States and Canada." Dunn, Peter A. Co-published simultaneously in *Journal of Housing for the Elderly* (The Haworth Press, Inc.) Vol. 12, No. 1/2, 1997, pp. 37-53; and: *Shelter and Service Issues for Aging Populations: International Perspectives* (ed: Leon A. Pastalan) The Haworth Press, Inc., 1997, pp. 37-53. Single or multiple copies of this article are available for a fee from The Haworth Document Delivery Service [1-800-342-9678, 9:00 a.m. - 5:00 p.m. (EST). E-mail address: getinfo@haworth.com].

INTRODUCTION

Housing adaptations are one of the key supports which enable older people to remain in their own homes and lead more independent lives (Gutman & Blackie, 1986). Modifications such as grab bars, handrails and ramps can assist elderly people to be more self-sufficient in their homes (Sherwood, 1981), enable them to get outside and be more active in the community (Dunn, 1990a) and even help in reducing the likelihood of institutionalization (Ratzka, 1984). However, policies and programs which promote accessible housing in many countries have been insufficient, uncoordinated and not very comprehensive. This paper will examine the need for barrier-free housing for elderly people in the United States and Canada, contrast the policy models which have been formulated in these countries and discuss a future framework for policy development. The United States and Canada were selected for analysis because, despite many similar needs of elderly people in these adjacent countries, two distinct policy models have evolved in these countries. This paper will compare the housing rights emphasis of the United States with the social welfare approach in Canada (Anderson, 1989).

Recent research studies have indicated the potential social and economic benefits of adapted housing (Chollet, 1979; Sherwood, 1981; Ratzka, 1984; Dunn, 1990a). Although the potential benefits of housing adaptations may be substantial, home modifications can often be made at a very reasonable cost. Project Open House, a program which adapts housing in New York City, spent an average of only $1,500 in 1986 to adapt existing homes of their clients. In fact, research has indicated that older people often require only small adaptations such as handrails and grab bars which are relatively inexpensive (Dunn, 1990a). The costs of adapting housing prior to construction are even less expensive than retro-fitting homes. In addition, units can be constructed to be "adaptable" to the individual needs of residents. For example, doors and corridors can be made wider, counters adjustable and bathrooms designed so that grab bars can be easily installed. Adaptable housing can be constructed so that everyone can use this universal design and the adaptation features are blended in inconspicuously.

A substantial number of elderly people in both the United States and Canada require barrier-free housing. Struyk (1982) found in his analysis of data from the 1978 U.S. Annual Housing Survey that out of 15 million elderly-headed households, approximately 8.6 million (57%) had a major health problem or mobility limitation. He estimated that approximately 1 million elderly households still needed housing adaptations. Dunn (1990b) determined in his analysis of data from the 1986 Statistics Canada's Health and Activity Limitation Survey that out of the 2.7 million elderly persons in Canada living in the community, 1.03 million (46%) had a physical, developmental or mental disability. Canada has a population approximately one-tenth of the United States. Roughly 33% of the 191,000 disabled elderly persons in Canada who required housing modifications did not have them. Although these surveys were undertaken at different times and utilized different definitions of disability and methods of calculating needs, they reveal that there is a sizeable number of elderly people in both countries who are disabled and require barrier-free housing. For the purposes of this paper, barrier-free housing will be considered as housing which is accessible and adapted to the individual needs of a person with a disability.

POLICY ISSUES

It is important to consider different housing policy approaches which can be undertaken to respond to this sizeable need. Donald Chambers (1986) explains that it is essential to consider the most effective form of benefit or service delivery when responding to a policy concern. However, he indicates that many social policies must pursue their objectives through multiple instruments or methods because of the complexity of social policy issues. In order to ensure a barrier-free housing environment for older people, several policy issues must be addressed. Housing policies must be developed to promote barrier-free housing in existing housing, new construction and rehabilitation. These policies may be different for private, public or non-profit housing as well as for single family homes or multi-unit construction. There are a number of other issues in formulating comprehensive barrier-free housing policies. For example, policies may have to deal with multiple jurisdictional levels of government and may need the support of public, private and voluntary sectors. In addition, the effective implementation of policies is also very important. Even the most progressive barrier-free guidelines can be problematic, if not implemented effectively.

Given the complexity of these issues, there are several policy approaches or options which government, non-profit and private organizations have undertaken to create barrier-free housing for elderly people. These policy options include: (1) Government Housing Construction Programs: national, regional or local governments can help finance or directly construct new housing for older people which is barrier-free including funding private, non-profit and/or cooperative housing agencies to develop new accessible housing; (2) Housing Vouchers: organizations can provide vouchers or certificates for elderly people to obtain and to pay for existing adapted housing units; (3) Community Service Approach: agencies can assess the housing needs of their clients and adapt existing housing units for qualified clients; (4) Grants, Loans and Reimbursements: government agencies can provide grants and loans directly to homeowners, tenants and/or landlords to adapt existing dwellings or health care insurance organizations can reimburse consumers for adapting their existing homes; (5) Building Codes and Regulations: different levels of government can ensure that new housing is barrier-free through enacting building codes and regulations; and (6) Human Rights Legislation: governments can establish legislation that prohibits discrimination against people with disabilities and requires that housing accommodate their disability. Figure 1 adapts a general matrix developed by Chambers (1986) to classify these policy options for barrier-free housing.

THE UNITED STATES RESPONSE

The United States has undertaken a number of different approaches which create more barrier-free housing. One of the major U.S. responses has been the financing of public housing for the elderly. These programs have increasingly emphasized barrier-free units, so that individuals can age in place. For example, the U.S. Department of Housing and Urban

FIGURE 1. Policy Options for Barrier-Free Housing

Policy Options	Forms of Benefit or Services
1) Government Housing Construction	Material Goods
2) Housing Vouchers and Certificates	Vouchers
3) Community Service Approach	Expert Services
4) Grants, Loans and Reimbursements	Cash
5) Building Codes and Regulations	Legal Regulations
6) Human Rights Legislation	Positive Discrimination

Development (HUD) has paid for the construction and some of the operating costs of public housing units for people with low incomes. These public housing projects are operated by over 3,300 local public housing authorities throughout the U.S. The local housing authorities provide housing in some projects for people of all ages; some projects have certain units designated for the elderly and some projects are entirely for elderly people. By 1990 there were 1.2 million federally supported, low-rent public housing units which were occupied, and approximately 40% or 482,000 units had elderly tenants (Special Committee on Aging, 1991). However, only about 25,000 new public housing units were constructed from 1986 to 1990 including 11,000 units for the elderly. Federal funding for the construction of new public housing units has virtually ended (HUD, 1990).

HUD's loan and assistance programs have been the major instrument for developing housing for elderly and handicapped persons. The Section 202 Direct Loan Program, which began in 1959, is HUD's primary program for producing housing for the elderly. This program has provided loans to community based non-profit organizations to construct or rehabilitate housing for the elderly. From 1974 to 1990, approximately 226,000 units were constructed for elderly people under this program. However, this program has been dramatically reduced with only 40,000 units being constructed from 1986 to 1990. HUD also operated the Section 231 and 236 programs which provided mortgage insurance programs for people with low incomes including the elderly, but these two programs were terminated in 1974. Approximately 66,700 units were constructed for elderly people under Section 231 and 82,170 units under Section 236. In addition, the Section 221 Mortgage Insurance Program for Multi-family Housing has created 155,734 units for elderly tenants of all incomes. Since 1981 HUD has dramatically reduced its budget for new construction. Section 202 is virtually the only new construction program currently being funded by HUD, albeit on a greatly reduced basis (HUD, 1990). In response to the dramatic decrease in federally sponsored housing programs, some state governments have created a range of innovative and cost-effective housing options for older people such as congregate housing, home equity conversions and homesharing.

There is no available data about what percentage of the federally sponsored housing units are barrier-free. However, in 1968 Congress passed the Architectural Barriers Act which required that federal government construction be accessible. The Rehabilitation Act of 1973 created the Architectural and Transportation Barriers Compliance Board under Section 502 to enforce this law and also required under Section 504 that all existing and new federally-funded programs be accessible in both the public and private sectors. Initially, HUD referred developers to the ANSI standards for accessibility, then HEW guidelines and then the Uniform Federal Accessibility Standards. However, it took HUD 15 years to finalize and publish its own requirements for Section 504 which requires that at least 5% of all federally-funded housing be accessible for people with mobility limitations and that 2% of housing be accessible for people with visual and hearing impairments. In addition to these overall regulations which HUD adopted to respond to civil rights legislation, regulations have been formulated for specific programs such as the Section 202 program.

Since the early 1980s, HUD has placed increasing emphasis upon housing subsidies and vouchers for elderly people, rather than constructing new housing for the elderly. The Section 8 Existing Housing program includes a certificate program which pays the difference between 30 percent of a tenant's income and the fair market rent. Older people can use the Section 8 certificate program to seek an affordable barrier-free housing unit. In 1983, a housing voucher program was created which is similar to the certificate program; however, the actual rent is negotiated by the tenant and landlord and the amount of subsidies are more limited. The tenant receives 30% of their income for rent regardless of the actual cost of the rent. In 1990, approximately 945,000 units were reserved for the certificate program and 250,000 for the voucher program. Roughly 46% of the certificate program funds were for elderly or handicapped individuals. Advocates of the certificate and voucher systems feel that these programs will avoid segregation and warehousing of poor people and allow individuals choices; however, others argue that there is already a critical shortage of housing for elderly people; landlords just increase rents because they know that tenants have additional funds available and very few new barrier-free housing units will be created through these demand-sided programs (Special Committee on Aging, 1990).

In addition, government and non-profit agencies adapt homes of disabled people. However, these approaches are piecemeal at best. Many of these community services have been geared primarily to assist younger adults to live more independently, to get out of their homes and to be employed. These programs are often not based upon individual need, but upon the category of service for which an individual qualifies. For example, individuals who qualify for the Veteran's Administration program might obtain renovations up to $35,000, while someone with similar needs on Medicaid might have few or no adaptations covered under this program (Dunn, 1986). In addition, some agencies provide small repairs and modifications using funds from the Older Americans Act for home supports (Hyde, 1989).

Grant, loan and reimbursement programs are even more sporadic and piecemeal in the United States. The U.S. does not have a comprehensive national grant and loan program which provides money for people to adapt their homes, even for individuals with low or moderate incomes. One exception is the Farmers Home Administration program which may provide low interest loans to rural homeowners aged 65 and over (up to $80,000) and grants (up to $5,000) for needed home adaptations. Some states such as Massachusetts have provided low-interest deferred loans to low-income homeowners through state bonding agencies for home repairs and adaptations. In addition, municipalities such as New York City and Oakland, California have used federal Community Development Block Grants for this purpose. Nevertheless, most elderly people are not covered by these programs (Dunn, 1986). Health care reimbursements such as Medicare do not fund home adaptations, although they will cover the expenses of durable medical equipment such as wheelchairs and walkers. Medicaid provides a broader response of reimbursements than Medicare. Several states have used the Medicaid waiver provisions to cover some housing adaptations although these programs vary considerably between the states. These adaptations must be cost-effective and reduce the need for a more restrictive, or costly setting. Private insurance companies with a few exceptions typically do not pay for adaptations and only if "its use is consistent with the insurer's obligations of maintaining/restoring a beneficiary's health and is perceived to be cost-effective" (Hyde, 1989, p. 4).

States may enact building codes to regulate the standards of new housing. States have gradually adopted barrier-free housing standards for new multiple unit construction or renovation projects. Usually building plans are approved for accessibility before construction. However, a 1979 survey found that state standards were very different and specific administrative and enforcement methodologies were often ineffective. Some architects might technically comply with state regulations, but because many architects are not committed to accessibility, these modifications are often inadequate (American Bar Association, 1979).

The policy approach which has recently had a major impact upon making present and future housing accessible in the United States is disability rights legislation. The 1973 Vocational Rehabilitation Act and its amendments established the framework for disability rights in the U.S. The Fair Housing Amendments Act (FHAA) of 1988 focused specifically upon housing discrimination and accessibility. It amended Title VIII of the Civil Rights Act of 1968 to add people with disabilities and families with children, so that they will not be discriminated against in terms of housing. From 1991, all new buildings with four or more units including public, private and non-profit housing have been required to be accessible according to new design criteria. This Act sets out specific design criteria including several adaptable housing features. Although this legislation is based upon individual complaints, it will also help bring state accessibility codes up to a national standard. States that wish to enforce these regulations and receive HUD funding for this purpose must legislate accessible state housing building codes which are at least substantially equal to FHAA's codes and regulations. The law also states that landlords must allow a person with a disability to make architectural modifications to an apartment (Disability Law Center, 1989). In 1990, the Americans with Disability Act (ADA) extended civil rights protection for people with disabilities in areas other than housing.

THE CANADIAN RESPONSE

In Canada, under the 1867 British North America Act, the responsibility for housing was delegated to the provinces. Because of this constitutional arrangement, it has been difficult for the federal government in Canada to initiate comprehensive barrier-free housing policies across the country. The federal government initiatives are embodied in the National Housing Act (NHA) and implemented by Canada Mortgage and Housing Corporation (CMHC). CMHC has chosen to influence housing through financial mechanisms such as grants, loans and insurance arrangements. CMHC has increasingly delegated these financial initiatives to the provinces in recent years (Gross, 1985).

From the inception, specific housing programs for the elderly were not singled out. In 1949 under the federal-provincial partnership agreement (Section 40), the federal government provided 75% of the capital and operating costs for public housing including housing for older persons, while the provincial and some municipal governments paid 25% of the costs. In 1964, the public housing program expanded rapidly when the federal government agreed to pay up to 90% of the capital costs (Section 43) and cost-shared operating expenses at 50-50 (Section 44) with the provinces and municipalities. However, the public housing program was discontinued in 1979 after constructing over 200,000 units, one-half of which were designated for the elderly. Partially because of the negative image of public housing, CMHC replaced this program with the Section 56.1 Social Housing Program. Under this program, CMHC provides insurance and subsidies to provinces and municipalities and non-profit organizations such as churches or co-operatives to construct non-profit units and co-operative houses including units for elderly people. The Social Housing program has been modified in recent years. Under the existing federal-provincial agreement the provinces can elect to administer any of these programs except the federal co-operative housing program which has been administered and financed by the federal government (Goldblatt, 1989).

Many of the earlier public housing units designated for elderly people were not fully adapted. Decisions regarding accessibility were primarily left to the provinces and local housing authorities. However, in 1981 in response to the International Year of the Disabled, CMHC began to require that at least 5% of all new federally financed units be accessible. CMHC has not yet adopted a policy of adaptable design for all units; however, CMHC is presently undertaking research in this field. There are approximately 250,000 federally funded elderly housing units. Roughly half are non-profit and co-op units and the balance are public housing stock. In the five years between 1986 and 1990, the Social Housing Program produced 46,524 units of which 19,573 units were for the elderly including 5,669 units which were modified for their needs (CMHC, 1991).

CMHC has instituted a rent supplement program which is cost-shared on a 75-25 basis with the provinces. The provincial governments subsidize specific units for lower-income recipients in non-profit, co-operatives, limited-dividend projects and in some private buildings. Individuals who receive rent supplements pay the same rents as they would in public housing. However, the Canadian government has not adopted a housing voucher or certificate system similar to the United States in which individuals seek out their individual housing unit (Gross, 1985).

Some provincial departments and non-profit organizations in Canada undertake minor housing modifications for their clients. However, this service approach is less emphasized in Canada than in the United States because of the fairly extensive federal and provincial programs which provide grants and loans for modifications to existing housing.

The real strength of the Canadian model is found in the federal and provincial grant and loan programs for disabled people to modify their existing housing. The federal Residential Rehabilitation Assistance Program (RRAP) was developed in 1973 as a general home improvement program for people with low to moderate incomes whose homes needed repairs and who lived in designated neighbourhood improvement areas. In 1981 this program evolved to include grants and loans for housing adaptations. In 1986, CMHC developed RRAP-D for disabled people with low to moderate incomes. This program provides individuals in need with a total of $10,000 in loans, including up to $5,000 in grants depending upon their income, to modify their homes. Individuals can also apply for RRAP funds for general renovations to their homes. From 1974 to 1990 the RRAP program helped renovate approximately 220,060 units, of which approximately 86,200 were homes of elderly people. Between 1986 and 1990, approximately 24% of 14,700 individuals who received loans and grants under the RRAP-D program were elderly people. CMHC also provided grants to landlords to make adaptations up to $5,000 for self-contained units and $2,500 per bedsitting unit, if the landlord brought the building up to standards and agreed to rent ceilings for 15 years. However, this program was discontinued in 1989 (CMHC, 1991).

Many of the provinces also provide grants and loans for home adaptations. Some of these programs were initiated to cover geographic areas which did not qualify for the earlier federal RRAP program. Some target certain groups in need such as elderly people who are frail. These programs provide a diversity of benefits from $350 to $15,000 to help people with home repairs and often with home modifications. For example, the Ontario Home Renewal Program for Disabled People (OHRP-D) was developed for people with disabilities regardless of income. Loans are provided up to $15,000 for home adaptations and all or a portion of this loan may be forgiven, dependent upon income (Ontario Ministry of Housing, 1986). It is important to note that despite Canada's extensive government health care system, most provincial health insurance programs do not cover housing adaptations, but they may cover assisted devices such as hearing aids, glasses, canes, walkers and wheelchairs.

Every five years the National Research Council (NRC) updates the National Building Code which acts as a guideline for the provinces as they revise their building codes for new construction and renovation of apartment buildings. In 1975 the National Building Code included accessibility requirements (Ontario March of Dimes, 1990). Nevertheless, according to the powers of the British North America Act, the provinces develop their own housing codes. The provinces of Newfoundland and Prince Edward Island do not have provincial building codes. Yet, the provinces have increasingly ensured that new apartment buildings are accessible. However, the extent of accessibility and adaptability varies between provinces. Generally, the provinces have established standards which ensure that private apartment buildings are accessible and that a certain percentage of units, usually 5%, are barrier-free.

The Canadian government has not developed extensive civil rights legislation for people with disabilities as in the United States. However, when Canada repatriated its Constitution from Britain in 1982, it established the

Charter of Rights and Freedoms. Section 15 of this bill of rights prohibits discrimination on the basis of mental or physical handicap. As a result, Canada is the first nation to have in their constitution a section prohibiting discrimination based upon handicap. Since this legislation was implemented, several far-reaching cases have been brought before the Supreme Court. These cases have expanded the protection of individuals with disabilities including older Canadians. Nevertheless, this Act has not been implemented into specific enforceable legislation such as the FHAA and ADA in the United States. Some disability advocates have prepared a federal omnibus bill which could amend existing pieces of federal legislation to incorporate anti-discriminatory provisions (Standing Committee on Human Rights, 1990). In addition, some of the provinces have revised their human rights codes to incorporate clauses prohibiting discrimination against disabled people in order to conform with the Charter of Rights and Freedoms. In 1989, Ontario led the provinces in establishing "Guidelines for Assessing Accommodation Requirements for Persons with Physical Disabilities," which allow individuals with disabilities to complain to the Ontario Human Rights Commission, if they do not feel that their environment adequately accommodates their disability, including their housing. Although these guidelines established major rights, these provisions primarily depend upon individuals to initiate complaints (Ontario Human Rights Commission, 1989).

DISCUSSION

The policy responses in the United States and Canada are similar in some respects, but also represent very different models which reflect different ideologies and jurisdictional arrangements in these countries. Both countries have emphasized the importance of housing options for seniors with different needs and the increasing role of state and provincial governments. Barrier-free requirements have been instituted in both countries for new publicly-financed housing including accommodation for elderly people. However, the U.S. has increasingly moved into a demand-sided voucher system and out of financing new construction even for elderly people. In addition, HUD's budget was dramatically reduced by 57% from 1980 to 1987, including basic programs for rental assistance for elderly and handicapped persons (Schwartz, Ferlanto & Hoffman, 1988). Therefore, despite progress in implementing barrier-free requirements for new public housing, there are far fewer new barrier-free units being constructed in the United States for elderly people. In contrast, CMHC continued to fund the

construction of a considerable number of new units of elderly social housing through the 1980s.

Another major difference in the policy approaches in the United States
and Canada is that the U.S. has depended upon a patchwork of uncoordinated government and voluntary agencies to adapt existing homes. This
model is consistent with the emphasis in the United States upon voluntary
charitable services. In contrast, Canada has developed a national grant and
loan model in which disabled people with low to moderate incomes are
given funds to adapt their homes. This model is reflective of a British
universal social welfare tradition. However, neither country has significantly expanded their health care systems to cover home modifications.
Medicaid perhaps has been the most responsive program. Nevertheless,
home adaptations continue to be considered primarily as a housing service
and not as a mechanism to promote health and to reduce accidents and
eventual hospitalization of elderly people with disabilities.

Both countries have increasingly had their building codes modified to
include barrier-free design for new private multi-unit construction and
renovations. These codes are primarily formulated at the state and provincial levels. There are considerable variations in the codes within both
countries; however, the evolution has been towards a more unified national response. The United States has dramatically moved in this direction
with the Fair Housing Act Amendment which requires that all new multi-
unit buildings adhere to basic barrier-free guidelines, while Canada still
depends upon national codes which provinces may adopt on a voluntary
basis.

The strength of the U.S. model is the expansion of disability rights. The
FHAA has significantly expanded the role of the federal government to
not only ensure that federally-funded housing be barrier-free, but also to
cover private and non-profit apartment buildings and to prohibit any form
of housing discrimination against disabled people. It builds upon a system
of civil rights in the United States. Although the law operates upon a
complaint basis, many states are also ensuring that their building codes
comply with this legislation. Canada's civil rights legislation is not as
comprehensive or prescriptive. Although the guidelines adopted by the
Ontario Human Rights Commission are closer to the U.S. rights-based
legislation, these guidelines are just for Ontario and they do not prescribe
specific housing standards for accessibility which must be adopted in
building codes. Other provinces may follow Ontario's lead, but very diver-
gent regulations and coverage may be created across Canada. One of the
major problems of creating national accessibility legislation in Canada is

that its Constitution clearly delegates the responsibility for housing to the provinces.

The barrier-free housing policies which have been developed in the United States and Canada reflect the ideologies of these countries and jurisdictional arrangements. Despite specific actions of individuals and pressure groups, these housing policies have evolved to reflect prevalent national ideologies. The present federal policies in the U.S. are consistent with the anti-collectivist U.S. ideologies outlined by George and Wilding (1985) which emphasize a limited government role in providing services, the use of vouchers and voluntary services for the very needy and the promotion of individual rights. The Canadian policies reflect more of a reluctant collectivist ideology with a substantial role for government in providing services, including a safety-net in the form of housing adaption loans and grants to ensure homes are barrier-free.

CONCLUSIONS

There does not appear to be one policy option which can ensure a barrier-free housing environment for all disabled elderly people in need because policies must respond to several different types of housing. For example, civil rights legislation such as FHAA can dramatically affect new construction; however, this legislation cannot help poor individuals to renovate their own homes. Grant and loan programs or voluntary services have a greater potential for helping these individuals. Policy options for each housing sector must be carefully considered in relation to effectiveness, costs and the empowerment of consumers. These policies must effectively address existing housing, new construction, and rehabilitation in the private, public and non-profit sectors.

One overall approach that the author feels has considerable potential is to combine the strengths of both rights-based legislation and comprehensive social welfare programs with the concepts of universal adaptable design (see Figure 2). Strong rights-based legislation and regulations could be adopted at the federal and/or regional levels such as the FHAA. Such legislation could ensure a social right for disabled individuals to have barrier-free housing and to provide a framework for other policy responses. This legislation could require that all new accommodation be barrier-free with very specific enforceable universal design standards, ensure that tenants could modify their own units and that disabled people would not be discriminated against in terms of any housing issues. In addition, it is important that housing codes be established which emphasize adaptable/universal housing design for all new construction and reha-

FIGURE 2. A Comprehensive Policy Approach

=====

(COMPREHENSIVE HOUSING POLICIES)

1. **NATIONAL RIGHTS TO ACCESSIBLE HOUSING**
   (For Individual Issues and to Guide Policy)

2. **UNIVERSAL ADAPTABLE HOUSING CODES AND PROGRAMS**
   (For New Construction and Renovations)

3. **A NATIONAL COMPREHENSIVE HOUSING ADAPTATION PROGRAM**
   (For Existing Housing and to Act as a Safety Net)

(COMMUNITY INVOLVEMENT AND CONTROL)

4. **COMMUNITY INFORMATION ON HOUSING RIGHTS**
   (Information on Seniors' Rights and Programs)

5. **CONSUMER INVOLVEMENT IN SERVICES**
   (Involve Seniors in Policies, Housing Adaptation Services and
   Management)

=====

bilitation. Such adaptable housing codes can ensure that housing can be easily adapted to people's changing needs. It is also important to consider ways in which adaptable design can be incorporated into the construction of new family homes. More publically funded barrier-free housing must also be constructed for seniors, especially because of the limited supply of housing and the dramatically increasing elderly population. A national universal program could be established to modify existing housing of tenants as well as homeowners in public, private and non-profit housing. Consumer control and involvement should also be encouraged. Elderly people can play an important role along with architects and designers in developing the plans for any new housing construction or renovations of existing buildings. Finally, consumers need to be informed about existing programs and their rights. One of the major reasons why many older people do not take advantage of housing adaptation programs is that they do not know about these programs and cannot obtain contractors to modify their homes (Dunn, 1985).

One of the next steps for the United States is to place priority on developing a more comprehensive grant and loan program for disabled people to modify their accommodation. Perhaps the next practical step in the United States would be to expand the Medicaid and Medicare systems to cover the costs of housing adaptations. A more comprehensive approach would be to initiate a national grant and loan program funded by HUD. The recent U.S. National Affordability Act of 1990 could be amended to include a provision for home modifications. In Canada, housing rights legislation needs to be expanded for people with disabilities. Any new Canadian disabilities rights bill should address the development of a national barrier-free housing standard. National legislation or consistent provincial legislation which is negotiated between the provinces and the federal government must ensure universal adaptable housing design in all newly constructed housing units similar to the FHAA legislation.

Nevertheless, every country has its own unique issues, jurisdictional arrangements and ideological approaches to social policy development. Each country will have to build upon their strengths in order to develop effective and comprehensive barrier-free housing policies.

POSTSCRIPT

The information for this paper was gathered in 1990. Since that time there have been considerable changes in housing policies for the elderly, especially in Canada. Not only has Canada been dramatically affected by a worldwide recession, but the free-trade agreement with the United States has severely increased unemployment as many manufacturers have moved to the United States where minimum wages are lower and labour laws less strict. At the same time the federal and provincial governments have been cutting public spending in order to reduce corporate taxes and transferring taxes from corporations to personal and sales taxes, so that corporations can be more competitive with businesses in the United States (Hurtig, 1991).

Over the last few years, the federal Conservative government in Canada has been slowly reducing its commitment to social housing. However, in 1992 the Canadian federal government radically changed its policies by instituting a cap on the growth of all new social housing expenditures, including for the elderly. This policy has meant a reduction of approximately 20% in 1992 and 30% in 1993 for new housing commitments including RRAP-D, the national program of home modifications. In 1994 the federal government plans to freeze the social housing budget which will mean the end of the national housing modification program, and curtail funding for any new social housing in Canada, unless additional internal savings can be generated by CMHC. One positive development is that CMHC has implemented Home Adaptations for Seniors' Independence

(HASI) across Canada. This two-year demonstration program provides low income elderly people 65 years and older with up to a $2,500 grant to pay for minor housing adaptations. CMHC allocated grants to adapt 3,800 housing units of elderly people over these two years across Canada. However, this program may not be continued past March 31st, 1994, depending upon the outcome of an evaluation and whether or not CMHC can generate any internal savings to pay for this program (CMHC, 1993).

In terms of barrier-free housing, there have been less changes in the United States than Canada in the last two years. Dramatic cutbacks in federal housing expenditures in the United States occurred ten years before those in Canada. Very little new federal housing for the elderly is being constructed in the United States. However, more states are using Medicaid waivers to cover housing modifications for the elderly. Plus, reverse mortgages are becoming more widespread for the elderly, so that they can take out some of the equity in their homes to modify their premises.

With the present ideology of cutting back government expenditures in both countries, a housing rights model may become increasingly useful in Canada as well as in the United States. Housing rights legislation can require that existing as well as new housing be barrier-free. Nevertheless, both countries need to construct more new barrier-free housing units for the elderly and provide a national housing adaptation program for existing homes in order to create an effective national barrier-free policy response.

REFERENCES

American Bar Association. (1979). *Eliminating environmental barriers: A statutory survey.* Washington, D.C.: U.S. Department of Health, Education, and Welfare.

Anderson, R.W. (1989). Comparing Canadian and U.S. approaches to creating accessible housing. Unpublished paper prepared for the Biennial Meeting of the Association for Canadian Studies in the United States.

Canada Mortgage and Housing Corporation. (1991). Special data provided to Dr. Peter Dunn by CMHC. Ottawa: Canadian Mortgage and Housing Corporation.

_____. (1993). CMHC. Housing Budget. Ottawa: Canada Mortgage and Housing Corporation.

Chambers, D. (1986). *Social policy and social programs.* New York: McMillan Publishing Company.

Chollet, D.J. (1979). *Cost-benefit analysis of accessibility.* Washington, D.C.: Department of Housing and Urban Development.

Disability Law Center. (1989). *The rights of persons with disabilities to be free from discrimination in housing pursuant to the federal fair housing law and other federal statutes*. Washington, D.C.: National Association of Protection and Advocacy Systems.

Dunn, P.A. (1986). *An analysis of housing adaptation programs in Massachusetts*. Boston: Adaptive Environment Center.

_____. (1990a). The impact of housing upon the independent living outcome of individuals with disabilities. *Disability, Handicaps and Society*, 9(1), 137-150.

_____. (1990b). The economic, social and environmental obstacles which seniors with disabilities confront in Canada. *Canadian Journal of Community and Mental Health*, 9(2), Fall, 137-150.

George, V. & Wilding, P. (1985). *Ideology and social welfare*. Boston: Routledge and Kegan Paul.

Goldblatt, S. (1989). Housing for seniors. *Perception*, 13(1), Winter, 25-28.

Gross, L.P. (1985). Federal housing programs. In G. Gutman and N. Blackie (Eds.), *Innovations in housing and living arrangements for seniors*. Burnaby, British Columbia: The Gerontology Centre, Simon Fraser University.

Gutman, G. & Blackie, N. (1986). *Aging in place: Housing adaptations and options for remaining in the community*. Burnaby, British Columbia: The Gerontology Research Centre, Simon Fraser University.

Hurtig, M. (1991). *The Betrayal of Canada*. Toronto: Stoddart Publishing Company.

Hyde, J. (1989). Summary of issues regarding reimbursement for home adaptations. Boston: Unpublished paper for the Adaptive Environments Centre.

Ontario Human Rights Commission. (1989). *Guidelines for assessing accommodation requirements for persons with disabilities*. Toronto: Ontario Human Rights Commission.

Ontario March of Dimes. Barrier-free Design Centre newsletter, Winter, 1988.

Ontario Ministry of Housing. (1986). *Access to building and facilities for disabled persons*. Toronto: Ontario Ministry of Housing.

Ratzka, A. (1984). *The costs of disabling environments*. Stockholm: Swedish Council for Building Research.

Schwartz, D.C., Ferlanto, R.C., & Hoffman, D.N. (1988). *A new housing policy for America*. Philadelphia: Temple University Press.

Sherwood, S. (1981). *An alternative to institutionalization*. Cambridge, MA: Ballinger Publishing Company.

Special Committee on Aging, United States Senate. (1990). *Developments in aging*. Washington, D.C.: U.S. Government Printing Office.

Standing Committee on Human Rights and the State of Disabled Persons, Canada House of Commons. (1990). A consensus for action: The resources for integration of disabled persons. Ottawa: Supply and Services, Canada.

Struyk, R. (1982). *The demand for specially adapted housing by elderly-headed households*. Washington, D.C.: The Urban Institute Project Report 3014-1.

U.S. Department of Housing and Urban Development. (1990). Special data provided to Dr. Peter Dunn from HUD Office of Budget. Washington, D.C.: Department of Housing and Urban Development.

Chapter 5

Accommodating the Elderly:
Words and Actions in the Community

Stewart Page

SUMMARY. The stigmatizing effects of the "elderly" label in obtaining community accommodation were examined, in a sample of 120 individuals advertising rooms or flats for rent in two Canadian cities, Windsor and London, Ontario. Telephone enquiries were made by an adult male (two conditions), young adult female, and an elderly (female) individual, who were ostensibly in search of rental accommodation. Rooms were significantly more likely to be described as unavailable when the caller was elderly, or when enquiries were made on her behalf. Comparisons are made to similar previous research and to current perspectives about community reactions to stigmatizing conditions. *[Article copies available for a fee from The Haworth Document Delivery Service: 1-800-342-9678. E-mail address: getinfo@haworth.com]*

The effects of a stigmatizing label or characteristic have been investigated increasingly ever since the classic research on psychiatric stigmatization by Goffman (1961) and by Amerigo Farina and associates (e.g., Farina, 1981) at the University of Connecticut. The issue of community

---

Stewart Page, PhD, is affiliated with the Department of Psychology, University of Windsor, 401 Sunset, Windsor, Ontario, Canada N9B 3P4.

[Haworth co-indexing entry note]: "Accommodating the Elderly: Words and Actions in the Community." Page, Stewart. Co-published simultaneously in *Journal of Housing for the Elderly* (The Haworth Press, Inc.) Vol. 12, No. 1/2, 1997, pp. 55-61; and: *Shelter and Service Issues for Aging Populations: International Perspectives* (ed: Leon A. Pastalan) The Haworth Press, Inc., 1997, pp. 55-61. Single or multiple copies of this article are available for a fee from The Haworth Document Delivery Service [1-800-342-9678, 9:00 a.m. - 5:00 p.m. (EST). E-mail address: getinfo@haworth.com].

55

acceptance of stigmatized persons continues to be of theoretical interest to social scientists (e.g., Breggin, 1991; Page & Day, 1990; Schellenberg, Keil, & Bem, 1995; Weiner, 1993) and the issue, of course, is also of practical importance.

As a result of educational efforts by the psychiatric and medical establishments (Page & Day, 1990; Sarbin & Mancuso, 1970; Weiner, 1993), it is no doubt true that persons with stigmatizing conditions are somewhat better accepted today. Yet, the frequent reliance upon data from "reactive" measures (Webb, Campbell, Sechrest, & Schwartz, 1966), that is, measures which are likely to distort the data which they elicit, continues to obscure the effects of stigmatizing conditions as these occur in everyday life. "Social distance" measures of stigmatizing conditions (Bogardus, 1959), which measure the degree of intimacy or social contact an individual indicates he/she is able to tolerate vis-à-vis another person ("I would not mind renting my house to . . ."), and so on, have been investigated by way of surveys or questionnaires. In these measures, the respondent indicates (e.g., says or writes) what his or her behavior would be in a given situation. Stigmatization has been far less frequently investigated, however, in actual social situations.

The issue of community accommodation is a significant factor in assessing the degree to which stigmatized persons are truly accepted. As one way of assessing this type of acceptance, the method of investigating availability of publicly advertised rooms or flats (apartments) was used widely during the early American civil rights movement. It was frequently found that rooms which were described as available, that is, when prospective tenants were White, were frequently described as unavailable when prospective tenants were Black. Using this method, Page (1977, 1983, 1995) found that unrented rooms, advertised in Toronto, Windsor, and Detroit newspapers, were almost always described as having been rented when telephone enquiries were made by callers who were ostensibly former psychiatric patients seeking accommodation in the community. Page (1989) also found that although 74 per cent of a sample of landlords in three Canadian cities (Windsor, Toronto, and Halifax) indicated in a telephone survey that they would be willing to rent rooms or flats to "AIDS patients," most described their rooms as being unavailable when telephoned enquiries were made by individuals who made brief references to themselves as indeed being such patients.

Using two Canadian cities, the present study explored the use of the telephone method to investigate the effects of the "elderly" label. As background, the present study is relevant to the earlier claims of Crocetti, Spiro, and Siassi (1974) that stigmatizing conditions (such as mental illness and, by implication, other types of stigma) no longer elicit discriminatory behavior in the community.

METHOD

Participants

Using four different conditions, as described below, calls enquiring about rental status were placed to a total of 120 landlords advertising (both furnished and unfurnished) rooms or flats, in two Canadian cities, that is, Windsor and London, Ontario ($N = 4 \times 15 = 60$ calls in each city).

Procedure

Advertisements were drawn from classified sections of the Windsor *Star*, and London *Free Press* newspapers. Procedures used were essentially the same as those described in previous research, cited above. No landlord, except in cases of no answer or busy signal, was contacted more than once, and only those including telephone numbers in their advertisements were contacted. Unless time or other restrictions were present in the advertisement, all enquiries were made in late morning or early afternoon hours, using the most recently available editions of the newspapers involved. As in previous studies, no call proceeded unless the person in charge of renting the room or flat, and/or someone who could give a definite (i.e., positive or negative) response regarding rental status, had been reached. Advertisements containing specific conditions, or preferences for prospective tenants, were excluded.

All calls were kept as brief as possible, generally of only several seconds' duration, and were limited to direct enquiries and initial responses only; that is, individuals were not prompted or asked to explain or elaborate their responses beyond indicating whether the room or flat was presently available. "Available" was defined as meaning that no firm rental arrangement had been made with another person. In previous research, simple enquiries regarding availability, following the above procedures, have located "still available" rooms from 90 to 100 per cent of the time.

In the first condition, the caller was an elderly female, 86 years old, possessing a characteristically "elderly" manner and voice. At the appropriate time, the caller said "Yes, uh, could you tell me, is the room advertised in the newspaper still for rent?" Upon receiving a substantive response, the caller said "OK, thank you," and ended the call.

In the second condition, the caller followed the above procedure. This caller was a young adult female, 20 years old.

In the third condition, the caller was an adult male.

In the fourth condition, the caller was an adult male, who indicated that he was making the rental enquiry on behalf of an elderly person who was in search of accommodation in order to "try things on her own for a while."

RESULTS

Data for both cities were pooled together. Goodness-of-fit (chi-square) analyses were performed on the frequencies of positive and negative responses concerning room availability in each condition. In each case, the degree of association between the frequency of positive and negative responses, and type of caller, was examined.

Table 1 shows the frequencies of positive and negative responses for each condition.

A chi-square test of the frequency data shown in Table 1, over all conditions, was significant, X^2 (3, $N = 120$) = 34.61, $p < .0001$. A chi-square (goodness-of-fit) test of the data for condition one only, involving the elderly caller, was significant, X^2 (1, $N = 30$) = 4.80, $p < .03$, as was that for the data in condition four only (male adult calling for elderly mother), X^2 (1, $N = 30$) = 6.53, $p < .011$. In these two cases, the proportions of positive versus negative responses were thus significantly different. As in previous similar studies involving enquiries made to several Canadian cities, and to landlords in Detroit, Michigan, no differences according to city, or gender of landlord, were found.

DISCUSSION

The fact of being elderly, or of having enquiries made ostensibly on behalf of an elderly person, significantly decreased the likelihood of a

TABLE 1. Positive and Negative Responses in Four Conditions (N = 120)

	Positive	Negative
Elderly Female	9	21
Young Adult Female	25	5
Adult Male	24	6
Adult Male (for Mother)	8	22

room or flat being described as available. The results are generally consistent with findings from similar studies cited above, including that of Page's (1989) study of ostensible AIDS patients seeking accommodation. From another perspective, the findings may not be totally consistent with Weiner's (1991, 1993) analysis of stigmatizing conditions. In this analysis, and probably also in "common sense" theory, the general public is assumed to be least likely to derogate or discriminate against persons with stigmatizing conditions over which they are believed to have little or no personal control or responsibility. However, while the elderly of course have no such control or responsibility, negative effects of the "elderly" label can and do still occur. The present data thus are also not consistent with the claims of Crocetti et al. (1974), that is, that stigmatizing conditions are no longer the occasion for discriminatory behavior in the community.

Social exchange theory (Thibaut & Kelly, 1959) holds that, in essence, individuals generally seek to maximize perceived rewards and minimize perceived psychological costs, in present or potential interpersonal situations. In contrast to results from surveys or questionnaires (which typically elicit high acceptance of stigmatized persons), many people in real life situations clearly choose to avoid the awkward or unfamiliar, as well as whatever hassles may be perceived as inherent in situations involving potential interaction with a stigmatized individual. It remains for future research to determine whether these facets of human nature, which operate in a different domain from that assessed by reactive questionnaires and social distance measures, are amenable to modification by educational efforts. In the meantime, it would appear that, despite increased knowledge and sophistication about the elderly in society, persons identified as elderly still face the prospect of rejection–at least when such rejection is privately expressed, seemingly "legitimate," and likely to be assumed by its perpetrator to be hidden and undetectable. The use of "low profile" or unobtrusive measures, as described by Webb et al. (1966) many years ago, thus remains valuable in identifying consistencies and inconsistencies between the domains of attitudes and behaviors, that is, between what people say and what they do. Updated knowledge of these differences should assist those studying both the effects of modern educational programs designed to increase community acceptance of stigmatized individuals. In the present perspective, it should be important to identify community situations in which the general public's accepting attitudes toward the elderly or other stigmatized persons may not be consistent with its private reactions and behaviors (Martini & Page, 1996; Weiner, 1993). For example, Page's (1989) previous study with telephoned landlords (cited above) found that most (74 per cent) said they would have "no problem" with the possibility of renting a room to someone with AIDS. Yet, the landlords' actual behavior, assessed unobtrusively, was largely inconsistent with their verbalized position.

It is acknowledged that the present study, and previous similar ones, used a research scenario which was somewhat contrived. The scenario is perhaps not relevant to the housing situations of many elderly individuals. Yet, the primary goal in its use was not the manifest issue of room availability per se, but rather the latent issue of the participants' underlying disposition toward the concept of the "elderly person" and the matter of its stigmatizing properties. The present sample of landlords, facing a situation in which personal contact with a caller appeared to be the likely result of a positive (room available) response, but in which they were able to decline help or involvement seemingly without detection (describing the room as unavailable), thus showed more behavioral rejection than acceptance. Clearly, in the case of the present elderly caller, this rejection was based only on the characteristics of the caller's voice and general manner. In the case of the male caller calling on behalf of the elderly person, it was seemingly based only on the landlord's anticipation of interaction with an elderly person.

Evaluation techniques or community programs aimed at assessing community attitudes toward the elderly, or persons with other stigmatizing conditions, must take account of the difference between the ideal and the real. In the writer's opinion, future research–possibly again following the general spirit of a "sting" operation–would be particularly valuable vis-à-vis important groups such as landlords or employers. Of course, other types of living situations, and their potential for acceptance and possible discriminatory actions, should be part of such research. The attitudes (perhaps, more importantly, the behaviors) of these important, nonstigmatized, groups would seem particularly critical as indicators of genuine community acceptance or rejection.

AUTHOR NOTE

Additional information regarding procedures or analyses may be obtained from the author upon request, or may be found in Page (1977, 1983, 1989, 1990). The author's mother served as the caller in condition one.

REFERENCES

Bogardus, E. (1959). *Fundamentals of social psychology.* New York: Century Press.
Breggin, P. (1991). *Toxic Psychiatry.* New York: St. Martin's Press.
Crocetti, G., Spiro, H., & Siassi, I. (1974). *Contemporary attitudes toward mental illness.* Pittsburgh: University of Pittsburgh Press.

Farina, A. (1981). Are women nicer than men: Sex and the stigma of mental disorders. *Clinical Psychology Review, 23*, 45-50.

Goffman, E. (1961). *Asylums*. New York: Anchor Books.

Human Rights Act. World Wide Web: http://nz.com/nz/queer/human.rights.html

Martini, T., & Page, S. (1996). Attributions and the stigma of illiteracy: Understanding help seeking in low literate adults. *Canadian Journal of Behavioural Science, 28*, 34-46.

Page, S. (1977). Effects of the mental illness label in attempts to obtain accommodation. *Canadian Journal of Behavioural Science, 9*, 85-90.

Page, S. (1983). Psychiatric stigma: Two studies of behaviour when the chips are down. *Canadian Journal of Community Mental Health, 2*, 13-20.

Page, S. (1989). Renting rooms in three Canadian cities: Accepting and rejecting the AIDS patient. *Canadian Journal of Community Mental Health, 8*, 53-61.

Page, S. (1995). Effects of the mental illness label in 1993: Acceptance and rejection in the community. *Journal of Health and Social Behavior, 7*, 61-80.

Page, S., & Day, D. (1990). Acceptance of the "mentally ill" in Canadian society: Reality and illusion. *Canadian Journal of Community Mental Health, 9*, 51-61.

Sarbin, T., & Mancuso, J. (1970). Failure of a moral enterprise: Attitudes of the public toward mental illness. *Journal of Consulting and Clinical Psychology, 82*, 268-280.

Schellenberg, G., Keil, J., & Bem, S. (1995). Innocent victims of AIDS: Identifying the subtext. *Journal of Applied Social Psychology, 25*, 1790-1800.

Thibaut, J., & Kelly, H. (1959). *The social psychology of groups*. New York: John Wiley.

Webb, E., Campbell, D., Sechrest, L., & Schwartz, R. (1966). *Unobtrusive measures*. Chicago: Rand McNally.

Weiner, B. (1991). Metaphors in motivation and attribution. *American Psychologist, 46*, 921-930.

Weiner, B. (1993). Sin versus sickness: A theory of perceived responsibility and social motivation. *American Psychologist, 48*, 957-965.

Chapter 6

Post-Occupancy Evaluation
of a Life-Care Community
for the Aged in Israel

Naomi Carmon

SUMMARY. This paper presents an advanced housing arrangement for elderly people and an innovative method of Combined Post-Occupancy Evaluation to evaluate it. The method is based on what we developed and found to be a useful checklist of housing-related needs–physical-functional and psycho-social–of elderly people. According to our findings, the fulfillment of the psycho-social needs has first priority in determining the satisfaction of the elderly with their environment. The evaluation method combines a two-fold professional evaluation and an evaluation by the users. The results of the evaluation lead to several practical recommendations, including a recommended reduction of the resources devoted to public areas in old-age homes and an increase of the investments in the individual housing units, in which most of the needs of the residents are fulfilled. *[Article copies available for a fee from The Haworth Document Delivery Service: 1-800-342-9678. E-mail address: getinfo@haworth.com]*

Naomi Carmon, PhD, is Head of the Graduate Program of Urban and Regional Planning, Faculty of Architecture and Town Planning, Technion–Israel Institute of Technology, Haifa 32000, Israel. E-mail: arrnc02@technion.technion.ac.il
This paper draws on empirical work done by Tamar Eyal-Elimelech as partial fulfillment of the requirements for a degree in Urban and Regional Planning at the Technion–Israel Institute of Technology, under the guidance of the author.

[Haworth co-indexing entry note]: "Post-Occupancy Evaluation of a Life-Care Community for the Aged in Israel." Carmon, Naomi. Co-published simultaneously in *Journal of Housing for the Elderly* (The Haworth Press, Inc.) Vol. 12, No. 1/2, 1997, pp. 63-81; and: *Shelter and Service Issues for Aging Populations: International Perspectives* (ed: Leon A. Pastalan) The Haworth Press, Inc., 1997, pp. 63-81. Single or multiple copies of this article are available for a fee from The Haworth Document Delivery Service [1-800-342-9678, 9:00 a.m. - 5:00 p.m. (EST). E-mail address: getinfo@haworth.com].

INTRODUCTION

The number and proportion of elderly people in the general population of every developed country is increasing steadily. Most of these people are able to function independently and continue to live within the communities where they spent their adult years. However, together with the increasing rise in life expectancy, there is a concomitant number of households with elderly people who need special living arrangements, because of problems of health, widowhood and/or social isolation.

Living arrangements have a significant effect on human behavior and quality of life (Cooper-Marcuse, Sarkissian and Sarkissian, 1986; Michelson, 1970). If this is true of regular people, it applies all the more to the elderly, who spend most of their time in or near their homes (Churchman, 1991). This is particularly true of elderly people who live in one form or another of housing intended specifically for senior citizens, since their arrangements are very often similar to those of a total institution. A total institution is defined as a formally managed residential site with a large number of people who are separated from the general population over a long period of time and share the life of a closed society (Goffman, 1961: XIII). For people who spend most of their time in such a closed environment, it is highly important to achieve the greatest possible congruence between their needs and the ability of their physical surrounding to fulfill those needs (French, Cobb and Rodgers, 1974; Kahana, 1982). According to Hoglund (1982), the needs which must be accommodated are, first of all, the physiological and functional needs of the aged person, followed by his/her psychological needs, especially independence and privacy, and finally, the needs of those who care for the elderly.

In order to ensure this congruence, many papers have been published which propose guidelines for design in conformity with the requirements of the elderly. Among the more interesting of these are Koff (1977), Howell (1980), Raschko (1982), who compared American, Canadian, German and Swedish standards, Patterson-Greer (1982), Zeisel, Epp and Demos (1983), Carstens (1985) and Valins (1988). Innovations in this field have recently been published by Regnier (1994).

Has the availability of many publications concerning housing for the elderly actually led to the creation of housing arrangements which fulfill the needs of the residents? A salient group of studies that were aimed at answering this question belong to the Post-Occupancy Evaluation (POE) school. This school developed in the 1960s and flowered in the 1970s and 1980s, gradually expanding beyond the confines of the universities to the province of professionals, attempting to devise solutions to practical problems (Knight and Campbell, 1980; Zimring and Reizenstein, 1980; Marans and Spreckelmeyer, 1982; Preiser, 1989). According to Grannis (1994), the POE has three characteristics: first, POE researchers approach the work of evaluation from the perspective of the occupant; second, POEs are prepared within the context of real-life settings after the home has been occupied for some time; and third, POEs are now generally prepared for a particular client with the goal of solving specific problems, rather than for the purpose of advancing or testing a theory.

Preiser et al. (1988) identified three different levels of POE–indicative, investigative, and diagnostic. Grannis (1994) explains the levels as follows: Indicative POEs, the simplest form, require only a few hours to a few days to complete. One of the most frequent applications of this level is to identify and correct minor problems in a new facility or design. The evaluation may consist of a review of building service records, interviews with staff members or the facility manager, and a personal walk-through inspection of the facility–typically conducted by an evaluator familiar with the particular settings. Investigative POEs are typically employed to determine underlying causes that give rise to more serious problems, and to suggest possible solutions. The information collected and the analyses made in the investigative POE are more detailed than those of the indicative POE and frequently involve specific evaluation criteria based on knowledge of the facility type, user group, organizational goals, and the explicit intent of the project. Diagnostic POEs are the broadest and most advanced form of evaluation. While indicative and investigative POEs are typically problem-oriented and site-specific, diagnostic POEs are designed to contribute to the state of knowledge about a facility or design product type. They require more sophisticated techniques of data collection and analysis and may take a year or more to complete.

One example of a diagnostic Post-Occupancy Evaluation is the work of Preiser, Rabinowitz and White (1988) on a senior citizens' center in Albuquerque. Before the center was built, an extensive literature review helped to determine the major goals of the facility, the activities considered in the design, and the potential future needs of the facility. Four existing centers were evaluated to ascertain what worked well in the facilities and what did not. The design recommendations that resulted from this evaluation process included improved lighting, circulation and lounge areas, and the designation of a meeting area with easy access to an outdoor space. The evaluation was used to develop a program for a specific center and also to develop a generic program for future senior citizen centers (Preiser and Pugh, 1986).

This article reports on a research project that integrates different levels of Post-Occupancy Evaluation and advances the state of the art by putting forth the following research goals:

1. To propose an advanced method of Post-Occupancy Evaluation for old-age homes which:

   - is related to a substantiated list of physical-functional and psycho-social needs of the elderly;
   - combines professional evaluations of the building with the evaluations of its occupants.

2. To apply the proposed method to an appropriate old-age home.
3. To use the analysis to draw generic (even though preliminary) conclusions for improved planning and design of old-age homes.

THE OBJECT OF THE EVALUATION: LIFE-CARE COMMUNITY FOR THE AGED

There are many typologies of housing for the elderly (see, for example, the list compiled by Eckert and Murrey, 1984). Shtarkshal (1978) identifies three basic forms, arranged in ascending order of support:

- Individual housing—the housing units are scattered throughout the community and the elderly occupants use the services available in the community; within the units, there are design elements and other facilities adapted to the physical limitations and safety requirements of the elderly residents.
- Congregate (sheltered) housing—assembled housing for independent elderly residents and those who are somewhat limited; each elderly person has his/her own home and may maintain an independent household, but auxiliary services for household management, maintenance, emergency assistance, etc., are available within the complex and are used by each resident according to need and wish.
- Long-term institutional care—residence in an institution which provides housing and support services for elderly people who cannot or do not wish to maintain an independent household.

This general list omits the most recent and sophisticated development in housing for the elderly (Wilder, 1994), which includes all three types of the following housing arrangements in a single complex:

- Self-contained houses/apartments, together with communal facilities which provide meals (for those who choose this option) and social activities.

- Personal care accommodations–usually in the form of single or double bedrooms and places where the elderly can receive assistance in eating, bathing, using of the toilet, etc., according to their needs.
- Nursing home facilities–similar to the personal care accommodations, with the additional availability of medical supervision and care.

In this configuration, the complex is both an institution and a community, but its image varies according to its physical components. Where the complex is composed of a relatively large number of scattered houses and buildings, it has the image of a community; where it is concentrated in one or a very few buildings, it has the image of an institution. In all cases, at least half–and frequently more–of the residents are independent elderly people.

This kind of life-long housing arrangement for elderly people was the object of our empirical research. Because this kind is designed for the most part for the middle class, we decided to investigate a middle-class place. For budgetary reasons, the investigation was limited to one complex only. The home selected was the Mozes home for senior citizens. This is a 30-year-old building, that contains all the above-mentioned housing arrangements for independent and frail elderly people. It is located in the heart of the Baka residential neighborhood of Jerusalem. Its population was suited to the research requirements: almost all of the residents were middle-class people who had a common cultural background; they immigrated to Israel in their youth, most of them from Central Europe and a few from Eastern Europe. This homogeneity enabled us to focus the discussion on the planning aspects of the old-age home, while minimizing bias stemming from the intervention of cultural variables, which cannot be controlled in a small sample.

HOUSING-RELATED NEEDS OF ELDERLY PEOPLE

We have taken as our point of departure the "environmental docility" proposition, according to which, as competence decreases, behavior is increasingly determined by exterior factors (Lawton et al., 1984). Appropriate housing arrangements for elderly people should therefore be based on a high level of congruence between the needs of the residents and the design of their surroundings (Marans et al., 1984). To achieve this, the planner and designer must have a comprehensive list of the housing-related needs of the target population. The development of such a list was among our research goals.

The research began with a literature survey. We found lists of basic human needs, lists of environment-related needs (among them: Murray,

1938; Maslow, 1954; Spivak, 1973; Kahana, 1982), and partial attempts to identify the special housing-related needs of the elderly (for example: Byerts and Conway, 1972; Brody, 1977; Poon, 1980; Carstens, 1985; Hoglund, 1985). We used all of these to compile our initial list, and divided it into two main parts: physical-functional needs (what people, including old, frail people, need in their environment in order to live as full a life as their physical health permits) and psycho-social needs (what they need in order to be satisfied with their environment).

With this initial list we approached ten professionals in the field of gerontology: social workers, designers and two managers of old-age homes. They all answered a "partly structured" questionnaire related to the comprehensiveness of the list and to the places in which the needs should be accommodated. These places were divided into three main areas of activity: within the private residential unit, within public spaces of the residential complex and its grounds, and outside this territory. Their answers were used to complete the final list that is presented in Table 1.

THE COMBINED POST-OCCUPANCY EVALUATION METHOD

Earlier post-occupancy evaluations of old-age homes were presented either a professional judgment (Osterberg, 1981) or the users' points of view (Duffy et al., 1986). We are proposing a combination of the two. The combined post-occupancy evaluation method developed for this research consists of a two-fold professional evaluation (the first two items below) and an evaluation by the users of the building, as detailed below:

- *Evaluation by compliance with professional standards and/or planning guidelines*–Most of the guidelines for planning of residential units for the elderly and public spaces in old-age homes, as well as the majority of standards for dimensions evaluated in this paper, were based on Israeli standards compiled by Valdman (1981). Guidelines connected with planning of outdoor areas and elements related to visual esthetics and safety, and part of those related to planning of public spaces outside the residential units were taken from Patterson-Greer (1982). With regard to the few details which were missing, in our view, from these two sources, standards were taken from other sources mentioned above. The degree of compliance with these guidelines was evaluated, based on observations and measurements in and around the building.
- *Evaluation by professional judgment*–The fulfillment of each physical-functional and psycho-social need in the old-age home and its

surroundings was evaluated by an architect with experience in the design on old-age homes and an experienced social worker. The architect relied on observations made at different times of day and night, in private apartments and in public areas in the selected complex, as well as in areas outside it, in order to relate to each of the needs that an old-age home is expected to fulfill. The social worker of the home was interviewed and requested to express her opinion concerning each of the same items.

• *Evaluation by the users*–Users were interviewed by means of a structured questionnaire which contained 150 questions, of which almost all were of the "closed" type (that is, with a few alternative answers determined in advance). The questionnaire was tested in a pilot study, changed, shortened and adapted to the research requirements and its population. The questions were related to demographic information concerning the interviewees, their behavior in the building, especially the frequency of use of its various spaces and services, and their opinions regarding the physical design elements, especially the degree of satisfaction with the areas allotted and the function of the various facilities. The questions were arranged to seek users' response regarding the fulfillment of each need on the above-mentioned list.

EVALUATION OF THE MOZES OLD-AGE HOME IN JERUSALEM: SELECTED FINDINGS

The Mozes old-age home is located at the heart of a middle-class neighborhood in Jerusalem. It is three stories high. The ground floor comprises the nursing section, which was not evaluated in this research. Elderly residents who function independently, as well as those who need some help in day-to-day functioning (but are not nursing patients), live on the second floor, which is actually the entry level of the building, and on the floor above it, which is reached by stairs or elevator. The research was aimed at the latter group and its housing arrangements.

Each single elderly person and each couple has a separate apartment. The building has two wings, an old one and a new one, with stairs and an elevator in each. The two wings are connected by a common entrance lobby. The old wing has 47 apartments for single occupancy and 12 apartments for couples, while the new wing has 29 apartments for single occupancy. The building's public functions include the lobby, administration offices, a dining room and kitchen, a library (which doubles as a club

TABLE 1. Housing-Related Needs of Elderly People and the Appropriate Place to Fulfill Them

Physical-Functional Needs

Residence

- Sleeping[1]
- Eating[1,2]
- Bathing, use of toilet[1]
- Laundry[1,2]
- Hospitality[1,2]
- Storage[1]
- View of open space[1,2]
- Communication (telephone, computer)[1,2]
- Home activity (hobbies, writing, etc.)[1]

Physical security

- Protection against accidents[1,2,3]
- Protection against violence[1,2,3]
- Protection against "getting lost"[1,2]
- Climatic comfort[1,2]
- Protection against environmental nuisance (noise, contamination, etc.)[2,3]

Psycho-Social Needs

Autonomy

- Personal control of a defined area[1]
- A sheltered area for intimate activity[1]
- Possibility of maintaining desired life style (maintenance of order, hours of light and darkness)[1]
- Possibility of accepting an area of responsibility and/or participation in decision-making related to old-age affairs[2]

Expression of personal identity

- Personal control over dressing, furnishing and decoration[1]
- Choice among a range of activities[1,2]

Social contacts

- Relationships with other people[1,2]
- Relationship with the community[3]
  - Participation in community life
  - Contribution to the community

Security for the future

- Assurance of housing in case of declining health[2]

Expression of social standing

- Demonstration of status[1,2,3] through:
  - – Location of the building
  - – Composition of the population
  - – Appearance of building and equipment
  - – Appearance of hospitality areas

Activities and services

- Cultural and social activities[2,3]
- Creative leisure activity[2]
- Paid employment[2,3]
- Voluntary activity[2,3]
- Commercial services[2,3]
- Convenient access by foot[2,3]
- Transportation (public, private, special)[3]

Special services for the elderly

- Cleaning and maintenance[1,2]
- Special health services[2]
- Special design and installations for residents with limitations of movement, sight, spatial orientation[1,2]

- -

[1]Should be fulfilled within the individual residential unit
[2]Should be fulfilled in the public spaces of the old-age home and its yard
[3]Should be fulfilled in proximity to the old-age home

71

room), a lecture hall, hair dressing salon, infirmary and synagogue. The building is connected to four outdoor areas: a patio and garden at the entrance, a small garden at the end of the old wing, a patio next to the new wing and a yard at the nursing floor level.

There are three types of single-occupancy apartments, each of which has an average floor area of 19-22 square meters. These units include a central space which is used for sleeping, sitting and hosting, a tiny entrance area, kitchenette and bathroom; some of the units have balconies. A unit designed for occupancy by a married couple has an area of approximately 39 square meters and includes, in addition to the above, a sleeping area of 12 sq m and a more spacious kitchen. With the exception of a clothes closet and kitchen cabinets, all of the furniture belongs to the occupants, most of whom brought the furniture from their previous homes.

We interviewed 50 of the 93 independent occupants of the self-contained small apartments. The choice of interviewees was done in such a way as to include persons of different ages and gender, single people and married couples, occupants of apartments in both wings of the building. Contact with the interviewee was made with the assistance of the social worker or the administrator of the home. The interviews normally lasted 45-60 minutes.

The 50 interviewees included 40 women and 10 men. All of them understood the questions and answered them willingly. Two-thirds of them were from 75-85 years old and the others were 86 or older. Eleven of them were married and lived in apartments for married couples, while 39 were single. Approximately 60% had lived in the home for 1-5 years and about 25% had lived there for a longer time, while the others had moved in more recently. All of these elderly people came to the old-age home from their homes in the community, most of them from Jerusalem itself, frequently from older, established neighborhoods (such as Rehavia and Bet HaKerem). In the past, most of them had worked outside their households, usually as professionals, skilled workers, clerks or sales personnel. Three-fourths of them had at least one health problem (heart disease, bone deficiencies, problems with sight, etc.), and one-third suffered from two illnesses or more.

In the course of the evaluation, a few findings of interest appeared to differentiate groups in the home. We found, for example, that there was a tendency towards increased satisfaction among most of the people questioned which corresponded with increase in age and the length of time they had spent in the home. In our opinion, this increased satisfaction mainly reflected the idea that the people had become accustomed to the place and made their peace with their situation. These differences are not presented in the analysis below, because the subdivision of such a small number of interviewees did not produce statistically significant results. We have related, therefore, to the 50 interviewees as a single group of residents in the Mozes old-age home in Jerusalem.

The evaluation findings were arranged in the form of tables; each table was composed of four columns: the first indicated the need (physical-functional or psycho-social); the second showed the actual situation, in comparison with the standards and planning guidelines; the third presented the professional evaluation and the fourth–the evaluation of the interviewed residents. Because of the limitation of space, we are unable to present in this paper all of these findings. Interested readers can find them in Eyal-Elimelech (Hebrew, 1990, to be translated into English). Discussed below are the principal findings only, arranged according to the three areas of activity we identified: the private residential units, the public spaces in the building, and the environment surrounding the home for the aged.

Evaluation of the Residential Unit

The area of the unit for a married couple was almost double that of a single-occupancy unit in the researched old-age home (see Figures 1 and 2). In the double-occupancy unit, the sleeping area was separated from the living room and both were separate from the kitchenette, while in the single-occupancy unit, these separations did not exist. It was no wonder, therefore, that both the professional evaluation and the degree of satisfaction of the residents were higher with respect to the double-occupancy

FIGURE 1. A Housing Unit for a Single Person (22 sq m)

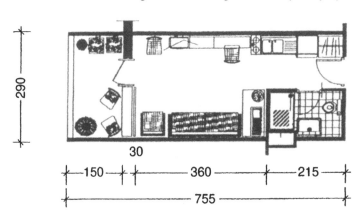

FIGURE 2. A Housing Unit for a Couple (39 sq m)

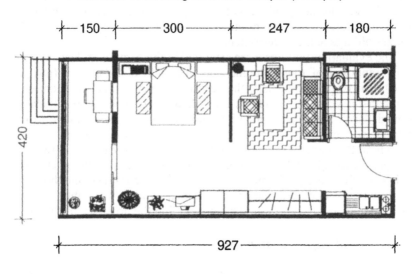

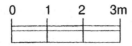

units. The surprising aspect was that, in spite of the small area of the single units (about 20 sq m, on the average), only 22% of the single residents maintained that they lived in "crowded" conditions, while all of the others said that the unit was "adequate," or even "roomy" (12%). Only one-third indicated the need for a separate bedroom; this was the case, despite the fact that half of those interviewed invited guests into their rooms, at least once a week. Only a few people complained about the size of the kitchenette, although many ate breakfast and supper in their rooms. Nor were there many complaints about the small bathroom. Only with regard to the lack of storage space were there many complaints from the residents, and 7 of them complained that they missed a balcony.

All of those interviewed, without exception, were satisfied with the maintenance of privacy which the apartments afforded them. Each resident had a his/her own apartment and the death of a partner did not obligate the survivor to relinquish the large apartment in favor of a small one. The regulations of the home prohibited staff from entering the apartments when their occupants were out, and when they were in, personnel might enter only after they had knocked on the door and been invited to enter. The residents appreciated the opportunity to furnish the rooms as they saw fit and only 4% were dissatisfied with the esthetic appearance of the apartments. All were pleased with the fact that each room contained a telephone with an outside line.

Evaluation of Public Areas in the Building

The evaluation by standards and design guidelines indicated that the planning complied, for the most part, with the recommended standards, in particular with respect to the lobby, sitting areas on the residential floors, balconies and gardens. The library in the elderly home was larger than required by the recommended standards, but the dining hall, lecture room, infirmary and laundry area were too small. In contrast with the standards, the home lacked clubrooms and commercial services (apart from the hair-dressing salon). The special design for protection against accidents and for assistance to the handicapped conformed to the standards.

In general, the professional evaluation was in agreement with the evaluation by standards, but it contributed a few additional details. It gave high points to the location of the lobby, the dining room and the sitting areas, as well as to the operation of the library and to the general form of the building. It included a detailed specification of the weaknesses of the dining room and recreation room and agreed with the evaluation by standards concerning the need for additional commercial services and a waiting room outside the infirmary. It emphasized a need for rooms for small group activities and additional public patios.

A decisive majority of the interviewees indicated a high degree of satisfaction with all of the services and public spaces provided for their use in the elderly home. Satisfaction was also expressed with regard to the security and safety arrangements in the building, the level of cleanliness and, especially, the existence of a nursing section, which gave a feeling of confidence with regard to the future.

However, great diversity was shown when it came to the degree of use by the residents of the various services and public spaces: the patio outside the new wing was spacious, attractive and well cared for; most of the residents praised the landscaping and care expended on it, but about 80% of them never used it and another 10% used it only "on rare occasions." Likewise, almost nobody visited the small garden by the old wing, even though its location was considered to be good by the professional evaluators and it was well protected from sun and wind and had suitable outdoor furniture. The spacious lobby, which was well divided into intimate areas, was the most frequented public space, but even here, 30% never used it and 40% sat there only infrequently. On the other hand, the recreation room was small and crowded, its location in the old-age home was considered to be unsuitable and its lighting and ventilation were insufficient; most of those interviewed complained that it was a stuffy room. In spite of this, 78% of the respondees said that they used its services at least once a week and frequently more often, especially to listen to lectures and concerts. Almost all of those questioned (95%) were satisfied with this service and the dual function of the room and saw no need for a separate club room.

Evaluation of the Environment Surrounding the Old-Age Home

The location of the building within a good residential area constitutes an important advantage, by any measurement. We found that the residents frequently used the nearby shopping center (82% made purchases there at least once a week), and a similar majority took walks through the neighborhood streets. All of those interviewed, without exception, expressed satisfaction with the possibility of reaching various parts of the city. About half of the residents used the transportation facilities, which were quite convenient, to go to a theater or a concert and many more went out to visit family and friends. About 10% worked at volunteer jobs outside the old-age home.

The planning guidelines call for participation by outsiders in the cultural and religious activities of an old-age home. Most of the residents were not in favor of this idea. Those of them who were religious were interested in opening the synagogue to the general public, because it was difficult to gather sufficient people from among the residents (a minimum of ten males is required for prayer in a synagogue). But the other activities–lectures, clubs, library, infirmary–most of the residents preferred to reserve for the permanent population of the old-age home. They were generally interested in expressing their ties with the community outside the home, rather than in it.

DISCUSSION AND CONCLUSIONS

With increasing life expectancy and significant increase in the population of the very old–75 years or over–the number of people who cannot or do not wish to maintain independent households is growing. Most of them, especially the more independent among them, do not have an appropriate housing solution, because almost all arrangements for long-term care—boarding homes, personal-care homes (domiciliary care), nursing homes, etc.–are designed for people with severe physical handicaps (for example, according to data presented by Lawton (1986: table 5.3) for residents of nursing homes in the United States, 86% were impaired in their ability to bathe and 58% were senile). For these mostly independent old persons, as well as for a smaller number of younger senior citizens, the solution of a life-care community seems to be most appropriate. It allows them a considerable degree of independence when they enter it, together with the highly important feeling of confidence that they will not be obliged to leave their environment in the future, even if they have to be (temporarily or permanently) nursing patients, or even if they become infirm. This kind of housing solution was the object of our research.

The conclusions drawn from this research are related to its method, to its modest contribution to theoretical understanding, and to its implications for the planning and design of old-age homes. An advanced method (a "diagnostic" analysis in the terms of Preiser et al. (1988)) of "combined post-occupancy evaluation" was successfully implemented in the empirical research. It was based on what we developed and found to be a useful and fruitful checklist of housing-related needs–physical-functional and psycho-social–of elderly people in a Western society, and it combined (a) a two-fold professional evaluation (by published standards and by on-site visits of professionals) of features in the building and around it; and (b) an evaluation by the users of the building. By shedding light from different directions on the various planning and design components, their advantages and disadvantages were disclosed.

Our findings support the theoretical proposition according to which the fulfillment of psycho-social needs has first priority in determining the satisfaction of people with their environment. People tend to be satisfied with the fulfillment of their physical-functional needs to a lesser degree, providing a higher degree of fulfillment of their psycho-social needs is available. Grandiose construction is not a precondition for satisfaction and certainly does not guarantee it.

The findings pointed at a limited space and several other physical disadvantages in the single-occupancy apartments, but these apartments fulfilled the psycho-social needs of their occupants almost to perfection; we assume that this is the reason for their very high degree of satisfaction with the apartments. Investigation of the public facilities revealed that it was not the size and convenience of a room which determined the extent to which it was used and the degree of satisfaction with it, but rather the nature of the service it provided, the quality of the service and its importance in the eyes of the interviewee. Of course, this does not mean that space and landscaping are unimportant. We found that the elderly took notice of elements in their physical environment, complained when they were unsatisfactory and praised that which they felt to be praiseworthy, but their order of priority between the physical and the psycho-social was clear.

Our research led to another conclusion related to the order of priorities: as with other ages, elderly people consider the individual domain to be more important than that of public spaces. The private apartment was depicted as the most important space for the residents, because it was there they spent most of their time and, apparently, fulfilled most of their needs. It is worthwhile emphasizing this conclusion, because it is not congruent with the recommendations of researchers/planners such as Howell (1980) and Ziesel et al. (1983), who attribute great importance to public areas adjacent to the apartments of the elderly, claiming that it is these areas which ensure social interaction. Nor does it conform to the generally accepted planning standards for the design of old-age homes (especially those located in a single building or a small number of buildings).

Accepted planning allots to public areas a very large portion of the total area and resources invested in the construction and equipment of old-age homes. We found that in the home we researched, 44% of the total area of the building was devoted to public areas, which is similar to several other plans of old-age homes we studied on other occasions. We also found that 70%-90% of the residents never, or only rarely used the gardens, public patios, lobby, or even the sitting areas on the residential floors; although the design of these areas was considered by both the professionals and the residents to be good, they were seldom in use. Hence, we recommend considering the possibility of a significant reduction in the resources devoted to such public areas. This subject should be investigated in other old-age homes, which have different populations with respect to age as well as their cultural, social and economic composition. If here too the findings are similar, the planning guidelines and standards will have to be adjusted. It will then be advisable to allot more space and resources to those functions which are used intensively, especially the individual residential units, and less to the public areas in general, especially those which are used rarely or almost not at all.

Other specific conclusions based on our research:

- The apartments, even if they are small, should be divided into separate spaces for daytime activities and entertaining company, sleeping, kitchenette and bathroom; a balcony, even if it is small, is important to many elderly residents.

- It is both possible and desirable to have public areas serve more than one purpose in order that they should be filled with activity during many hours of the day and week; a large room might be used as both library and club room, or as club room and place for prayer, according to the wishes and customs of the population.
- The desirable contact between the home and the community is outward-, rather than inward-directed; the residents were less interested in making the facilities of the old-age home available to the neighborhood in general, but did want easy access to the services of the community and the city.

The old-age home we investigated in this research was built thirty-five years ago. Its construction is not pretentious, but of good quality. Despite the general rise in accepted standards, it is a good home for its occupants even today, both according to the professional evaluation and the degree of satisfaction with it of the residents themselves. In our opinion, its main advantages, in order of importance, are: the provision of separate residential units for each single person and each married couple which include, in addition to living and sleeping space, a kitchenette, bathroom and private telephone; the existence of a nursing section within the complex; a close-to-homogeneous population; location within a "good" (middle-class) urban community, with easy access through organized transportation to all parts of the city; provision of services which are important to the specific population within the elderly home (in our case, these included lectures, concerts and a respectable library); and finally, good quality construction and design which gives a feeling of space and beauty to its occupants.

REFERENCES

Brody, E. (1977), *Long-Term Care of Older People*. New York: Human Sciences Press.

Byerts, T. and O. Conway (1972), *Behavioral Requirements for Housing for the Elderly*. Washington, D.C.: American Institute of Architects.

Carstens, Diane Y. (1985), *Site Planning and Design for the Elderly: Issues, Guidelines and Alternatives*. New York: Van Nostrand Reinhold Company.

Churchman, Arza (1991), *Housing for the Elderly and the Meaning of Home*. Haifa: Technion–Israel Institute of Technology, The Center for Urban and Regional Studies (Hebrew).

Cooper-Marcuse, Claire and Wendy Sarkissian (1986), *Housing As If People Mattered*. Berkeley, CA: University of California Press.

Duffy, Michael, Su Bailey, Bets Beck and Donald G. Barker (1986), "Preferences in Nursing Home Design: A Comparison of Residents, Administrators, and Designers." *Environment and Behavior*, Vol. 18 (2), pp. 246-257.

Eckert, J. Kevin and Marry Ittman Murrey (1984), "Alternative Modes of Living for the Elderly: A Critical Review." In Irwin Altman, M. Powell Lawton and Joachim F. Wohlwill (Eds.), *Elderly People and the Environment*. New York: Plenum Press.

Eyal-Elimelech, Tamar (1990), *Evaluating the Design of a Home for the Elderly*. Thesis submitted as partial fulfillment of the requirements for M.Sc. in Urban and Regional Planning, Faculty of Architecture and Town Planning. Haifa: Technion–Israel Institute of Technology (Hebrew).

French, J.R.P., Jr., S. Cobb and W.L. Rodgers (1974), "A Model of Person-Environment Fit." In G.V. Coelho, D.A. Hamburg and J.E. Adams (Eds.), *Coping and Adaptation*. New York: Basic Books.

Goffman, Erving (1961), *A sylums*. Garden City, NY: Doubleday.

Grannis, Peg (1994), "Postoccupancy Evaluation: An Avenue for Applied Environment-Behavior Research in Planning Practice." *Journal of Planning Literature*, Vol. 9 (2), pp. 210-219.

Hoglund, David J. (1985), *Housing for the Elderly: Privacy and Independence in Environments for the Aging*. New York: Van Nostrand Reinhold Company.

Howell, Sandra C. (1980), *Designing for Aging: Patterns of Use*. Cambridge, MA: MIT Press.

Kahana, E. (1982), "A Congruence Model of Person-Environment Integration." In M. Lawton, P.G. Windley and T.O. Byerts (Eds.), *Aging and the Environment: Directions and Perspectives*. New York: Springer Press.

Knight, Christopher R. and David E. Campbell (1980), "Environmental Evaluation Research: Evaluator Roles and Inherent Social Commitments." *Environment and Behavior*, Vol. 12 (4), pp. 520-532.

Koff, Theodore H. (1977), "Service Needs, Environmental Resources and Quality of Life: National Overview of the Elderly Population." *Journal of Architectural Education*, Vol. 31 (1), pp. 5-7.

Lawton, M. Powell (1986), *Environment and Aging*. Albany, NY: Center for the Study of Aging.

Lawton, M. Powell, Irwin Altman and Joachim F. Wohlwill (1984), "Dimensions of Environment-Behavior Research: Orientation to Place, Design, Process and Policy." In Irwin Altman, M. Powell Lawton and Joachim F. Wohlwill (Eds.), *Elderly People and the Environment*. New York: Plenum Press.

Marans, Robert W., Michael E. Hunt and Kathleen L. Vakalo (1984), "Retirement Communities." In Irwin Altman, M. Powell Lawton and Joachim F. Wohlwill (Eds.), *Elderly People and the Environment*. New York: Plenum Press.

Marans, Robert W. and Kent F. Spreckelmeyer (1982), "Measuring Overall Architectural Quality: A Component of Building Evaluation." *Environment and Behavior*, Vol. 14 (6), pp. 652-670.

Maslow, A.H. (1954), *Motivation and Personality*. New York: Harper and Row.

Michelson, Wiliam (1970), *Man and His Urban Environment: A Sociological Approach*. Reading, MA: Addison-Wesley.

Murray, H.A. (1938), *Explorations in Personality*. New York: Oxford University Press.

Osterberg, Arvid (1981), "Post-Occupancy Evaluation of a Retirement Home." *EDRA 12*, Proceedings of the 12th International Conference of the Environmental Design Research Association, Ames, IA, pp. 301-311.

Patterson-Greer, Julianna (1982), *Surpassing the Regulations: Building Superior Facilities for the Aged*. North Texas State University, Center for Studies in Aging.

Poon, L.W. (Ed.) (1980), *Aging in the 1980s*. Washington, D.C.: American Psychological Association.

Preiser, Wolfgang, Harvey Z. Rabinowitz and Edward T. White (1988), *Post-Occupancy Evaluation*. New York: Van Nostrand Reinhold Company.

Preiser, Wolfgang F.E. (Ed.) (1989), *Building Evaluation*. New York: Plenum Press.

Raschko, Bettgann Boetticher (1982), *Housing Interiors for the Disabled and the Elderly*. New York: Van Nostrand Reinhold Company.

Regnier, Victor A. (1994), *Assisted Living Housing for the Elderly: Design Innovations from the United States and Europe*. New York: Van Nostrand Reinhold.

Shtarkshal, Miriam (1978), *Sheltered Housing for the Aged–Planning Principles*. Jerusalem: Brookdale Institute for Gerontology (Hebrew).

Spivak, M. (1973), "Archetypal Place." In Wolfgang Preiser (Ed.), *Environmental Design Research*, 1:33-46. Stroudsburg, PA: Dowden, Hutchinson and Ross.

Valdman, Lee (1981), *Guidelines for Designing Old Age Homes in Israel*. Jerusalem: Eshel (Hebrew).

Valins, M. (1988), *Housing for Elderly People: A Guide for Architects, Interior Designers and Clients*. New York: Van Nostrand Reinhold Company.

Webster's Seventh New Collegiate Dictionary (1967), Springfield, MA: G. & C. Merriam Company Publishers.

Wilder, Madelyn (1994), "Housing for a Retirement Community." *Journal of Housing for the Elderly*, Vol. 11 (1), pp. 67-76.

Zeisel, John, Gayle Epp and Stephen Demos (1983), *Midrise Elevator Housing for Older People–Behavioral Criteria for Design*. Cambridge, MA: Building Diagnostics, for the US Department of Housing and Urban Development, Office of Policy Development and Research.

Zimring, Craig M. and Jonet E. Reizenstein (1980), "Post-Occupancy Evaluation: An Overview." *Environment and Behavior*, Vol. 12 (4), pp. 429-450.

Chapter 7

Housing the Rural Elderly:
A Place for Abbeyfield?

Bonnie C. Hallman
Alun E. Joseph

SUMMARY. This paper presents a case study of the potential of the Abbeyfield model of small congregate housing to meet the needs of the rural elderly. The results of interviews with thirty key informants indicate a very guarded assessment of Abbeyfield *despite* expressed dissatisfaction with current housing supply and options. Further analysis indicates a more favourable climate for Abbeyfield in smaller, more remote communities. Service producers/managers and municipal officials are more sceptical about Abbeyfield than are the elderly themselves, although these opinion leaders base their opinions upon assumptions about what the elderly want. We believe that these perceptions may be coloured by an experience of broken promises, failed experimentation and short-lived innovation. *[Article copies available for a fee from The Haworth Document Delivery Service: 1-800-342-9678. E-mail address: getinfo@haworth.com]*

INTRODUCTION

Our interest in age-segregated housing reflects the fact that housing for the elderly is patently more than shelter. As the point of access to the

Bonnie C. Hallman, PhD, and Alun E. Joseph, PhD, are affiliated with the Department of Geography and Gerontology Research Centre, University of Guelph, Guelph, Ontario, Canada N1G 2W1.

[Haworth co-indexing entry note]: "Housing the Rural Elderly: A Place for Abbeyfield?" Hallman, Bonnie C., and Alun E. Joseph. Co-published simultaneously in *Journal of Housing for the Elderly* (The Haworth Press, Inc.) Vol. 12, No. 1/2, 1997, pp. 83-103; and: *Shelter and Service Issues for Aging Populations: International Perspectives* (ed: Leon A. Pastalan) The Haworth Press, Inc., 1997, pp. 83-103. Single or multiple copies of this article are available for a fee from The Haworth Document Delivery Service [1-800-342-9678, 9:00 a.m. - 5:00 p.m. (EST). E-mail address: getinfo@haworth.com].

surrounding social and physical environment and as the locus for social exchange and consumption of services, "home" has a pervasive impact on the life quality of the elderly (Joseph and Martin-Matthews, 1993; O'Bryant, 1983). Housing also represents an important resource for communities attempting to cope with the needs of their aging populations (Joseph and Fuller, 1991). In turn, our interest in rural communities reflects their demographic status. About one in three elderly Canadians lives in communities outside the typical cityscape (Joseph and Martin-Matthews, 1993); and it is not uncommon to find individual rural communities with proportions of elderly population (65 years or older) exceeding 30%, with correspondingly high percentages of very old residents (80 years or older) (Hodge, 1991).

Our immediate point of departure in this research is the observation that rural communities and their elderly residents are typically and systematically disadvantaged in terms of their access to age-segregated housing (Gutman and Hodge, 1990; Hodge, 1987; Joseph and Fuller, 1991). Indeed, the initial objective of this paper is to characterize gaps and deficiencies in the provision of age-segregated housing in heterogeneous rural communities with elderly populations of different size and composition. This discussion of supply and demand establishes the context for a more specific exercise, the assessment of the potential of the Abbeyfield model of congregate housing to meet the needs of rural communities and their aging residents.

Our research emphasizes Canadian conditions and issues, and features a case study of rural communities in southern Ontario. Nevertheless, we believe that the issues we address are common to many jurisdictions in North America and that many of our results are similarly generalizable.

The remainder of this paper is composed of four major sections. We begin by considering the broad parameters of rural aging, stressing connections between aging patterns and the provision of age-segregated housing. This general discussion of rural aging and housing provides the platform for the section that deals with the design of the case study. Here, specific attention is paid to the nature of the Abbeyfield model and to the strategies and procedures employed in data collection. A further section presents the major results of the case study, emphasizing the assessment of the Abbeyfield model in light of the distinctive circumstances of communities. The paper concludes with an overview of results and a critical reconsideration of issues associated with the provision of age-segregated housing in rural communities.

GROWING OLD IN RURAL COMMUNITIES

Rural Population Aging

Population aging is one of the unifying features of rural regions across Canada (Hodge, 1987; Martin Matthews, 1988), and is usually measured in terms of the number of elderly people as a proportion of total population, which we refer to as "relative concentration." However, within most regions a "demographic divide" exists between *nucleated* rural communities with generally high, or very high, proportions of elderly in their total populations, and *dispersed* rural communities with markedly lower proportions of elderly (Hodge, 1987; Joseph and Martin-Matthews, 1993). For instance, in their study of Grey County, Ontario, Joseph and Cloutier (1991) report that towns and villages typically had proportions of elderly over 20% in the mid-1980s, while townships had proportions of elderly at or near the provincial average of 10.9%.

High levels of relative concentration of elderly persons in nucleated communities result, in part, from the movement of older persons out of neighbouring dispersed communities (Dahms, 1987; Joseph and Martin-Matthews, 1993). Thus, in any analysis of rural aging and its social ramifications, it is necessary to take a broad view of rurality that acknowledges such interconnections. Indeed, a good case can be made for maintaining that strong and diverse links exist between rural and small town Canada (Martin Matthews, 1988) and for considering settlements of less than 10,000 as distinct elements of the *rural* settlement system (Hodge and Qadeer, 1983; Hodge, 1987).

The distinct yet complementary nature of population aging in nucleated and dispersed rural communities has emerged strongly in research on rural housing and residential choice. The availability of age-segregated housing, and of amenities and services generally, underlies much of the net transfer of older persons from dispersed to nucleated rural communities (Hodge, 1984, 1987; Joseph and Fuller, 1991). These short-distance migrants swell the numbers of elderly persons aging in place in rural towns, where they may also be joined by long-distance migrants in search of small town living (Bowles and Beesley, 1991; Joseph and Cloutier, 1991).

However, it is unwise to overgeneralize the nature of population aging in nucleated rural communities. Hodge and Qadeer (1983) note that smaller rural towns, especially those with populations under 2,500, may not be well endowed with services, and this has implications for their ability to support expanding elderly populations. Strong regional differences are also apparent (Joseph and Martin-Matthews, 1993), and these may confound size effects. Moreover, within particular regions, rural towns proximate to (service-rich) urban centres will provide environments for aging quite distinct from those found in more isolated communities of similar size. In fact, this is all part of the diversity of the rural aging experience that has struck many commentators (Coward, 1979; Joseph and Martin-Matthews, 1993; Keating, 1991). Nevertheless, we believe that housing availability and residential choice provide useful means for generalizing about both the aggregate (community) and individual experience of rural aging.

At the aggregate level, we have noted already that the differential availability of age-segregated housing plays a part in promoting the accumulation of elderly persons in particular communities (e.g., see Joseph and Fuller, 1991). At the same time, it is evident that a supply of appropriate housing allows communities to cope effectively with the needs of their aging populations (Gutman and Blackie, 1984). In contrast, at the individual level it is residential choice, a behaviour that binds aging individuals to their communities, that is critical. Housing supply is a pre-condition for residential choice and is therefore an appropriate starting point for any analysis of their interconnection.

Housing the Rural Elderly

The supply of age-segregated housing in rural Canada has generally been characterized as "inadequate" (Gutman and Hodge, 1990; Hodge, 1987; Joseph and Fuller, 1991). The supply of institutional facilities such as chronic care hospitals and nursing homes, meanwhile, has generally been in line with legislated norms (Joseph and Martin-Matthews, 1993). However, the availability of various intermediate housing forms, such as congregate projects of various types, has been demonstrably less adequate (Joseph and Fuller, 1991; Nicholson, 1987). These intermediate housing forms are geared to seniors whose ability to remain living in the community is dependent upon limited assistance with tasks of daily living (Monk and Kaye, 1991). It follows that rural seniors in need of such supportive housing may often be faced by uncomfortable choices: "either 'struggling on' in inappropriate housing or accepting premature institutionalization in a local facility; or perhaps either staying on in a familiar community or moving to one that offers more suitable housing" (Joseph and Martin-Matthews, 1993, p. 8).

Seniors in need of intermediate, supportive forms of age-segregated housing are likely to be older, and to be widowed and female (Health and Welfare Canada, 1989). They are also likely to be socially isolated (Cape, 1987) and transport-dependent (Grant and Rice, 1983), and to be experiencing associated problems in accessing support services (Joseph and Fuller,

1991). This vulnerable group of elderly widowed women is the fastest grow-ing cohort in many rural communities (Joseph and Martin-Matthews, 1993).

Given the obvious need for intermediate forms of age-segregated hous-ing, why are they generally lacking in rural communities? To a great degree, the answer involves "numbers." While rural communities typical-ly display higher levels of relative concentration of elderly population than do urban centres, levels of (absolute) congregation are markedly higher in cities (Rosenberg, Moore and Ball, 1989). Cities present government agencies and other housing providers with large numbers of potential consumers in close proximity to each other. In contrast, while the elderly may constitute a high proportion in rural community populations, numbers are relatively small. Thus, the target population for seniors' housing may be larger and more obvious and accessible in urban areas.

A second impact of numbers of elderly in rural communities also re-lates to congregation, although in this instance the emphasis is on attain-ment of "threshold populations" for particular age-segregated housing proj-ects. Simply put, a given level of congregation does not translate smoothly into demand for a particular type of housing. The heterogeneity of rural elderly populations, manifested in contrasting life histories, circumstances and residential preferences, means that the potential market for age-segre-gated housing is fragmented (Golant, 1991; Gutman and Hodge, 1990), with the great majority of elderly wanting to stay on at home as long as possible (Bakiuk, 1990; Ontario Advisory Council on Senior Citizens, 1992). Combined with low levels of congregation, this fragmentation of the potential market for age-segregated housing has confounded attempts to expand residential choice for the rural elderly (Joseph and Fuller, 1991).

Responding to the simultaneous observation of housing inadequacy and market fragmentation, commentators have called for innovative, small-scale congregate projects catering to elderly rural residents in need of limited assistance (e.g., see Hodge, 1987; Joseph and Fuller, 1991). However, except for a study by Gutman and Hodge (1990), very little is known about the receptiveness of rural communities to particular types of congre-gate housing. The remainder of this paper is devoted to a case study of the potential place of the Abbeyfield model of congregate housing in rural southern Ontario.

THE CASE STUDY

The Abbeyfield Model of Congregate Housing

Congregate housing is ". . . a residential setting that is non-institutional, but adapted to meet the special needs of elderly persons through good design of the physical environment and the provision of some supportive services" (Cronin, Drury and Gragg, 1983, p. 1). Congregate housing may also be called "enriched housing," "sheltered housing" or "shared housing," and design philosophies and service provision may vary widely. However, ". . . whatever term and design used, the intent of a congregate program is to provide services in a residential setting for . . . persons who can no longer single-handedly manage the tasks of everyday living . . ." (Monk and Kaye, 1991, p. 8).

The Abbeyfield model of congregate housing originated in the United Kingdom more than thirty years ago, and it is now promoted by an international federation of volunteer-based local societies. The primary objective of each Abbeyfield Society is the provision of family-like accommodation for single elderly people (Shimizu, 1988). The essence of the Abbeyfield model is that it emphasizes lifestyle as much as shelter.

There are an almost infinite number of ways to describe any congregate housing project (Golant, 1991). In assessing the receptiveness of rural communities to the Abbeyfield model, we believe that primary consideration should be given to the description provided in the Abbeyfield promotional literature. This literature, which takes the form of pamphlets and handbooks, emphasizes seven aspects of the Abbeyfield model (see Shimizu, 1988):

- *Small scale*; family-like atmosphere promoted by having only 5 to 10 residents.
- *Active connection with the community*; the location of Abbeyfield Houses on "ordinary streets" allows residents to maintain contact with relatives, friends and the community at large.
- *A context of mutual and interdependent support*; the creation of an environment that is meant to foster care and enjoyment among residents.
- *A full-time resident housekeeper* (assisted by a part-time assistant); oversees meals and the general operation of the house, and is responsible for "making the house a home."
- *Private space for each resident*; residents have private bed/sitting rooms to complement communal living space.
- *Continuity*; provided through a support organization under the auspices of the local and national Abbeyfield societies.
- *Non-profit and financially self-sustaining*; this usually necessitates the support of churches or services clubs like Rotary.

Data Collection

To assess the potential of the Abbeyfield model of congregate housing for the elderly, data were collected in six rural communities in southern Ontario. Following arguments set out earlier in the paper (e.g., see Joseph and Martin-Matthews, 1993), the six communities were selected to represent two inter-locking aspects of rurality, namely population size and urban proximity. Following Hodge and Qadeer (1983) and Scheidt (1984), communities were selected to represent three size classes (1,000-2,499, 2,500-4,999 and 5,000-9,999). Additionally, communities were chosen to represent degrees of proximity and remoteness vis-à-vis the urbanized core of southern Ontario.

The locations of the six communities nominated for inclusion in the case study are shown in Figure 1, and summary demographic data are presented in Table 1. With the exception of Erin, a community known to have been strongly affected by residential growth generated within the Toronto-centred region (Smit and Joseph, 1982), each community displays a relative concentration of elderly persons that exceeds that for the province as a whole. Proportions of elderly are consistently higher in the more remote towns than in the three communities more proximate to the Toronto-centred region and to the cities of Guelph (population of 87,976 in 1991), Cambridge (92,772) and Kitchener-Waterloo (239,463) that lie at the southern boundary of the study area (Figure 1). At the same time, the relative concentration of the elderly in total populations generally *decreases* with community size. The proportion of the population aged 75 years or older also tends to be higher in smaller and more remote communities, although departures from the provincial norm are more extreme than they are for the population aged 65 or older. At nearly three times the provincial level, the relative concentration of the "older-old" is particularly notable in the more remote communities of Markdale and Durham.

In each community, baseline data on the local availability of age-segregated housing were accumulated from published sources and verified by a field survey. These data portray the objective circumstances of housing supply that constitute local constraints on housing choice. A second phase of the data collection involved a structured interview with a purposive sample of thirty key informants drawn from the six communities. The key informant approach was identified as an efficient means of tapping the opinions of 'constituencies' we considered relevant to the assessment of the Abbeyfield model.

The elderly themselves are the most numerous constituency whose opinion is important for the assessment of any innovation in age-segre-

FIGURE 1. Location of the Study Communities

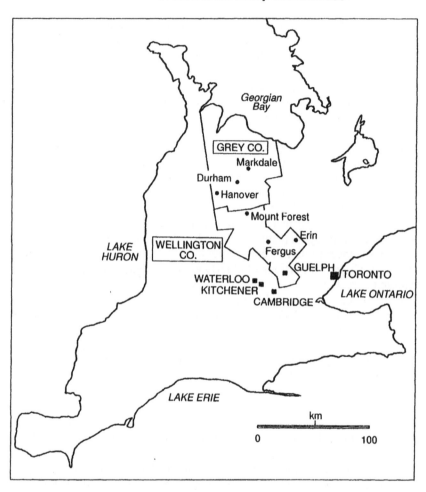

gated housing. Thus, it is not surprising that the elderly have been the *exclusive* focus of virtually all studies of rural housing demand and supply (e.g., see Gutman and Hodge, 1990). Yet it is also well accepted that individuals in positions of knowledge and authority may have a considerable influence on the success or failure of local initiatives. In the case of housing innovations in rural towns, we believe that housing and service managers/providers constitute knowledgeable people who can facilitate or

TABLE 1. Selected Demographic Characteristics of Study Communities (1991)

	Total Population	% aged 65 or older	% aged 75 or older
Markdale*	1,370	27.7	14.2
Erin	2,489	7.6	3.2
Durham*	2,558	25.2	13.3
Mount Forest	4,266	20.9	10.8
Hanover*	6,711	20.0	10.4
Fergus	7,940	14.2	6.8
Ontario	10,084,885	11.7	4.7

Note: * indicates communities classified as "more remote."

retard innovation. Municipal officials may play a similar role but may operate more from a position of authority than one of knowledge.

One municipal official was interviewed in each community, for a total of six key informants in this category. Two elderly residents known to be opinion leaders were interviewed in each of the four larger communities, and one each in the remaining two communities, for a total of ten. Two managers/providers were interviewed in each community, one each from the housing and service sectors, with an oversampling of providers in two communities, for a total of fourteen. In total, thirty interviews were carried out.

The interview schedule was structured according to guidelines set out in Feldman (1981) and Kushman and McClure (1985). The majority of questions were open-ended, although several pre-scaled questions elicited assessments of selected aspects of the Abbeyfield model. Questions were organized to lead respondents along a pre-determined path, from the general assessment of gaps and deficiencies in housing for the elderly, to a specific assessment of the potential for the Abbeyfield model in their community. Personal interviews were conducted in the summer and fall of 1990 and took from thirty minutes to two hours to complete, at an average of about one hour each.

RESULTS

The results of the case study are presented in three parts. Initially, we focus on the housing supply data which describe the objective circumstances that limit the residential options of seniors. Second, key informant assessments of gaps and deficiencies in *local* housing supply are presented. These subjective evaluations of local conditions are compared to the objective data, and form the backdrop for the presentation of key informant assessments of the Abbeyfield model.

Community Housing Supply

The supply of age-segregated housing in each of the six communities is shown in Table 2. Three major categories representing increasing levels of care provision are used: seniors' apartments, congregate homes and nursing homes. Within the seniors' apartments category, a distinction is made between public-sector developments, which attract subsidies and are available only to low-income seniors, and private-sector developments. Seniors'

TABLE 2. Supply of Age-Segregated Housing in Case Study Communities (1990)

	Seniors' Apartments		Small Congregate Homes (15 beds)		Congregate Homes		Nursing Homes	
	Projects	Units	Homes	Beds	Homes	Beds	Homes	Beds
Markdale	3	42	-	-	-	-	1	77
Erin	3	74	-	-	-	-	-	-
Durham	3	47	-	-	-	-	2	148
Mount Forest	5	105[1]	1	14	1	49	1	87
Hanover	4	155[2]	-	-	2	146	3	143
Fergus	2	69	1	4	1	42	1	62

Notes:
[1] 61 units are in private-sector developments.
[2] 100 units are contained in a single private-sector development.

apartments are not "serviced," which distinguishes them from congregate homes (variously referred to in southern Ontario as "rest homes," "retirement homes" and "lodges") that offer services ranging from meals to limited (up to 1 1/2 hours per week) nursing and personal care (Forbes, Jackson and Kraus, 1987). Given the focus of this research on a small congregate housing option, homes of less than fifteen beds are broken out within this category. Nursing homes provide extensive personal and nursing care (more than 1 1/2 hours per week) in addition to the residential function they share with congregate homes. Homes for the Aged, which have a tradition of separate funding and administration in Ontario, can be included under the Nursing Home category because of their functional similarity (Forbes, Jackson and Kraus, 1987). New legislation has already addressed differences in funding and accountability (Ministries of Health, Community and Social Services and Citizenship, 1993), and it is almost certain that the Ontario government will legislate a merger of these two long-term institutional care categories in the near future.

With the exception of Mount Forest, the communities with population under 5,000 offer extremely limited residential options to their aging residents (Table 2). Given that only low-income seniors can qualify for public sector apartments, for many elderly persons in Markdale and Durham, institutionalization is the only option to staying on at home. In Erin, options are even more limited. Among the smaller towns, Mount Forest is exceptional in the choice offered to its residents: public and private seniors' apartments, small and large congregate homes and a nursing home. A range of housing options is also available in the two largest towns, Fergus and Hanover (Table 2), although the latter has a larger total supply and offers more choice of facilities. Thus, the data support the notion of a positive relationship between community size and housing supply/residential choice. In contrast, the relationship of housing supply to urban proximity is less clear. In two of the size classes (1,000 to 2,499 and 5,000 to 10,000), the remote community offers more housing options than does the urban proximate community, but in the middle size class (2,500 to 4,999), the reverse is true.

The simultaneous manipulation of the demographic (Table 1) and housing data (Table 2) yields additional insights into the housing situation in each of these six communities. As shown in Table 3, the ratio of seniors' apartments to resident population aged 65 or older is generally in the range of 6 to 12 units per 100 persons, with Erin as a conspicuous outlier. In contrast, the combined ratio of congregate and nursing home beds to resident population aged 75 or older is in the range of 20 to 44 beds per 100 persons. These latter figures, which can be interpreted as estimates of

TABLE 3. Provision Rates of Age-Segregated Housing

	Apartment units per 100 persons aged 65 or older	Congregate beds per 100 persons aged 75 or older	Nursing home beds per 100 persons aged 75 or older
Markdale	11.1	-	39.5
Erin	38.9	-	-
Durham	7.3	-	43.5
Mount Forest	11.8	13.7	18.9
Hanover	11.5	20.9	20.4
Fergus	6.1	8.5	11.5

an "institutionalization rate," support the contention that the supply of housing plays an important role in promoting *local* congregation of the older elderly in rural towns.

In summary, the six communities provide an interesting window on the objective circumstances of housing supply in rural towns. There are strong effects associated with community size, such that larger communities offer a more varied and richer menu of housing options. Somewhat weaker effects are associated with urban proximity. It follows that the aging residents of some communities have greater residential choice than do their peers living elsewhere. However, it is important to acknowledge that the availability of local housing options does not guarantee accessibility. Places may *not* be available in the appropriate housing project at the right time *and* at the right price. Indeed, the fact that nursing homes are always subsidized, while rest homes are generally not, goes some way toward accounting for the popularity of the institutional option in Ontario (Forbes, Jackson and Kraus, 1987).

Local Perceptions of Housing Supply

Key informants were asked to indicate gaps and/or deficiencies in the local provision of age-segregated housing *and* to provide an assessment of consequent impacts on senior citizens in their communities. Nearly all saw a need for additional age-segregated housing in their communities. Municipal officials usually expressed a desire for "more of the same," especially seniors' apartments, but wanted better design to facilitate residents aging in place. A few elderly residents were of a like mind, but the majority did not identify *any* gaps or deficiencies in the local provision of housing for the elderly. In contrast, the majority of service managers/providers identified a local deficiency in *supportive* housing options geared to the elderly in need of limited assistance. As one provider respondent put it, 'There are not enough semi-independent options. We have residents who could be maintained in a more independent way.'

Whatever the prevalent supply conditions (see Table 2), the need for supportive housing was identified by some respondents (primarily service managers/providers) from all communities. However, in the two smallest communities in the study (Erin and Markdale), specific concerns about the lack of supportive living options were subsumed within a general concern about the lack of housing options for seniors. In the other communities, the gap in supportive housing was pinpointed more precisely.

In terms of the impacts on elderly residents of gaps and deficiencies in housing supply, there was a recurrent view that the elderly in rural towns have little room to manoeuvre. Many respondents noted the plight of seniors in need of limited assistance to maintain their independence. One key informant picked up on the theme of "leaving the community": 'Seniors have had to leave to find suitable housing if they need supervision or mild care.' Another noted the tendency for "premature institutionalization": 'I know of several people who have gone into homes. They really don't require care at this level . . . I wonder why they are there?' Among the key informants, service managers/providers were the most likely to identify impacts arising from the local (un)availability of housing options, although several municipal officials were also sensitive to the problems experienced by local elderly. Consistent with their reticence concerning gaps and deficiencies in housing supply, elderly residents were the least likely to identify impacts. Notwithstanding the similarity of concerns across all the communities, a closer examination of the interview transcripts indicated a tendency for assessed impacts to be viewed as profoundly adverse in more remote *and* smaller communities.

Assessments of the Abbeyfield Model

The assessment of the Abbeyfield model proceeded in two stages. Following a standardized description, key informants were asked to list the positive and negative features of the Abbeyfield model. Respondents were then asked to assess the *local* potential for Abbeyfield.

All the key informants had something positive to say about Abbeyfield. Not surprisingly, most of these comments mirrored the description of the model, and positive comments are replete with references to "privacy," "independence," "companionship," "a family atmosphere" and "sense of security." Notwithstanding this similarity in general comments, both service managers/providers and municipal officials tended to cite the continuance of community living as a prominent positive feature of the Abbeyfield model. In contrast, elderly residents did not take such a broad view of housing choice, opting instead to comment on possible financial savings for individual seniors.

The assessment of negative features of the Abbeyfield model was more diverse. At a general level, elderly residents unfamiliar with the model were concerned with its newness in Canada and preferred to put their faith in "tried and true" options. Service providers/managers and municipal officials voiced concerns about the availability of financial support for the development and operation of Abbeyfield Houses. One manager had an extremely negative view of the Abbeyfield model, noting that such intermediate housing forms might '. . . cheat seniors by giving them less than they could have. . . .' Other managers/providers and some municipal officials saw Abbeyfield as an expensive and inefficient alternative to small retirement lodges.

Apart from these contrasts between elderly residents', service managers/providers' and municipal officials' views of the Abbeyfield model, respondents were almost unanimous in their views of the resident compatibility issues associated with Abbeyfield. Some key informants pondered over the general difficulties of bringing together a small number of unrelated individuals to live in a "home-like" environment. Others were more specific, doubting the willingness of elderly people used to living alone to live with others, especially those of a different sex. In a related vein, a few respondents wondered if the only common factor among residents would be their advanced age, and others saw the prohibition on couples as a weakness of the model.

Assessments of the potential of the Abbeyfield model to meet the needs of *local* seniors are presented in Table 4. No key informants felt that the Abbeyfield model had "*very* strong" potential in their community. In the smaller communities (of less than 5,000 people), the modal response was "strong" potential, whereas in the larger communities it was "moderate" potential. It is notable that the three respondents who felt that Abbeyfield had no potential at all were from urban proximate communities. It is also of some interest that the five key informants who saw Abbeyfield as having little or no potential in their communities were service managers/providers or municipal officials. Elderly residents believed that Abbeyfield had either strong or moderate potential in their communities. As one

TABLE 4. Key Informant Ratings of the Potential of the Abbeyfield Model

Potential is . . .	Communities with Population < 5,000		Communities with Population > 5,000	
	#	(%)	#	(%)
Very strong	-	-	-	-
Strong	9	(47.4)	3	(27.3)
Moderate	7	(36.8)	5	(45.4)
Little	1	(5.3)	1	(9.1)
None	2	(10.5)	1	(9.1)
Undecided			1	(9.1)
	19	(100.0)	11	(100.0)

elderly resident put it, 'There is a need for more congregate housing, particularly in communities like this. Seniors want the intimacy of small groups.' This strong, positive sentiment contrasts with the reticence expressed when seniors were asked to consider gaps and deficiencies in housing supply.

When asked about the potential ease or difficulty of setting up an Abbeyfield House in their communities, the majority of key informants believed that it would be "somewhat difficult" (Table 5). In elaborating on their views, respondents described a conservative attitude amongst both local decision-makers and small-town seniors. This is manifested in reluctance to accept change; to "abandon the traditional" and adopt new ideas and concepts. As one manager/provider said, 'People in rural areas are slow to change. If something is developed locally, and they have confidence in the individual promoting it, it can fly–provided he's not a politician!' Additionally, many key informants commented on "resistance" among the elderly, not only to the introduction of new concepts but also to the reality of getting older. As one elderly resident put it, 'There is a resistance to aging in this community. People are very proud.' The existence of this attitude has been noted by other researchers (e.g., see Filion, Wister and Coblentz, 1992; Wister, 1989).

Key informants from smaller communities (less than 5,000 people) were somewhat more optimistic about the ease of establishing an Abbey-

TABLE 5. Key Informant Assessment of the Ease/Difficulty of Establishing an Abbeyfield House

Establishing a House would be . . .	Urban Proximate Communities		More Remote Communities	
	#	(%)	#	(%)
easy	-	-	1	(7.1)
relatively easy	1	(6.3)	1	(7.1)
neither easy or difficult	-	-	3	(21.4)
somewhat difficult	13	(81.1)	7	(50.0)
very difficult	1	(6.3)	-	-
undecided	-	-	2	(14.3)
not applicable[1]	1	(6.3)	-	-
	16	(100.0)	14	(100.0)

Note:
[1] This category was introduced post facto because one respondent was so negative about Abbeyfield that she refused to provide an assessment.

field House than were those from larger communities. However, urban proximity is the more dominant effect in these data, with all but one of the key informants from the urban proximate communities indicating that it would be difficult to establish an Abbeyfield House locally (Table 5). While service managers/providers were the most optimistic of the key informant groups, they also furnished the most extreme ratings, with one manager declaring that it was 'out of the question.'

DISCUSSION

The objective data on the supply of age-segregated housing in the six study communities paint a familiar picture of heterogeneous environments for aging (e.g., see Gutman and Hodge, 1990; Joseph and Fuller, 1991). Nevertheless, the data appear to support the contention that housing options increase with settlement size, such that larger towns offer a broader and richer housing menu (e.g., see Hodge, 1987; Joseph and Martin-Matthews, 1993). Although less dramatic, there also appear to be some effects associated with urban proximity, with more remote communities offering more options *locally.*

Regardless of these contrasts in the objective circumstances of communities, most of our key informants believed the local supply of age-segregated housing to be deficient. Most respondents, especially those in the larger communities, pinpointed a "gap" in the provision of supportive housing catering to elderly persons in need of limited assistance to maintain independence. Consistent with expectations expressed in the literature (e.g., see Joseph and Martin-Matthews, 1993), key informants in all communities cited premature institutionalization and pressure to leave the community as consequences of a local shortfall in age-segregated housing. This suggests that the supply of housing in our study communities should be thought of as indicative of varying levels of "deficit." Even in the best supplied community, judgements of adequacy are not favourable.

Service managers/providers were the key informants most likely to identify deficiencies in housing supply. Elderly residents seemed content with the status quo, an attitude that might be interpreted as yet another manifestation of rural stoicism (e.g., see Joseph and Fuller, 1991). We believe that a more fundamental reason for this preference for the status quo lies embedded in an almost universal preference to "stay put" (e.g., see Filion, Wister and Coblentz, 1992; Joseph, 1992).

Filion, Wister and Coblentz (1992, p. 21) note that ". . . elderly persons seem to display an aversion toward residential change. This is evidenced by high satisfaction with their present residence and an apparent lack of interest in housing alternatives." They go on to suggest that the elderly may be "adapting in place" as much as "aging in place." This mindset may promote the under-valuation of environmental difficulties and a consequent reluctance to acknowledge the need for alternative, age-segregated housing. As one of our manager/provider respondents put it, 'It's so hard to get seniors past staying in their own home. Most of our admissions come right from home, and the change was a big adjustment for them.' This preference for staying put also colours attitudes toward specific housing models like Abbeyfield.

When asked to comment on the positive and negative aspects of the Abbeyfield model, nearly all the key informants cited the basic attributes of Abbeyfield (small scale, supportive, etc.) as positive features, but they cited a *diversity* of negative features. Some of these concerns, such as the compatibility of residents, touch at the core of the Abbeyfield concept and therefore merit attention. Others, such as the concern that Abbeyfield does not cater to couples, relate more to a desire for a single housing model to meet the needs of all elderly; "to be all things to all (wo)men." Such concerns are difficult to address, but they do suggest the need for more careful explanation *and* justification of this, and other, housing models.

Perceptions of the Abbeyfield model translate into assessments of its potential to meet the housing needs of local seniors. Twelve of our thirty key informants felt that Abbeyfield had "strong" potential, while a further twelve felt that it had only "moderate" potential. The remaining six felt it had "little" or no potential or were undecided (Table 4). Service managers/providers and municipal officials dominated the negative group and came primarily from urban proximate and/or larger communities. In elaborating on their assessments, these managers/providers and municipal officials expressed a strong preference for "tried and true" alternatives, namely serviced apartments or conventional (large) congregate projects. They felt that, properly developed, such age-segregated housing forms could meet the needs of elderly persons in their communities.

Turning to the issue of the ease/difficulty of establishing an Abbeyfield House, the majority of respondents (who had seen strong or moderate potential for Abbeyfield in their community) became a little pessimistic. Twenty key informants felt that it would be "somewhat difficult." One manager was so negative that she refused to assess the ease/difficulty of establishing an Abbeyfield House. Respondents cited conservative attitudes in their communities and a basic reluctance to entertain options to aging in place as the reasons for their pessimism.

Looking across these results, it is interesting to note that community size and urban proximity do *not* fit easily into generalizations about the subjective assessments of housing deficiencies or the potential of the Abbeyfield model to fill a "gap." While, objectively-speaking, age-segregated housing is both more plentiful and more varied in larger communities, the likelihood of a key informant indicating need for additional housing was not clearly related to community supply conditions. In contrast, community size and urban proximity did have some role to play in determining assessments of the potential of Abbeyfield to meet local needs. These community attributes also affected perceptions of the ease/difficulty of establishing an Abbeyfield House. All in all, respondents from smaller, more remote communities saw some potential in the Abbeyfield model and were a little more optimistic about the ease of establishing a House locally.

On the whole, our results support the argument that the limited options facing people growing old in rural communities reflect the fundamental difficulty of supplying a variety of housing forms to a small and fragmented marketplace (e.g., see Joseph and Fuller, 1991). Our data also support the contention that the majority of seniors want nothing to do with *any* age-segregated housing form. Those who are willing to assess an alternative like Abbeyfield usually do so using the yardstick of their own home with its "past reality" built up over a lifetime. As Golant (1991) notes, this invariably results in poor assessments of congregate housing projects that have only a "present reality."

Our interviews also revealed a strong tendency for key informants to favour the familiar over the unfamiliar. This was also evident in Gutman and Hodge's (1990) study of the housing preferences of elderly residents in ten rural towns from three regions of Canada. They reported a strong and consistent preference for well-established forms of age-segregated housing. Our study extends their results, by noting that the bias toward the familiar is even stronger among service managers/providers and municipal officials than it is among the elderly themselves. It was this group of community-opinion leaders who were most sceptical about Abbeyfield. We believe that the absence of input from these groups constitutes a major deficiency in studies that have informed previous discussions of rural housing for seniors.

Above all, our results underscore the challenge of meeting the housing needs of the rural elderly. While the Abbeyfield model appears to the expert, outsider eye to have some potential in small and more remote communities, there are several hurdles that would have to be overcome to translate potential into reality. Education is clearly necessary. Potential elderly residents have to be "sold" on Abbeyfield. They have to be convinced that it is an affordable option and does not constitute institutionalization. Above all, they have to be convinced that Abbeyfield is a viable alternative to "staying put." Assuming that sufficient demand is established, local organizations and institutions have to be persuaded to "come on board." This is undoubtedly a difficult task; small rural communities in Ontario have always found it difficult to sustain volunteer-based activities (Joseph and Martin-Matthews, 1993). This negative experience of broken promises, failed experimentation, and short-lived innovation undoubtedly colours local perceptions of housing models like Abbeyfield.

To end on an optimistic note, we are encouraged that the more positive assessments of the Abbeyfield model and the greater optimism concerning the ease of setting up a House came from key informants in smaller, more remote communities. It is in such communities that, objectively speaking, the Abbeyfield model holds the greatest potential. The small number of seniors in need of supportive housing *and* interested in making a residential move means that small congregate housing projects are the only viable means of expanding housing choice in these rural communities.

REFERENCES

Bakiuk, E. (1990) "Exploring the Option to Age in Place." *Plan Canada* 30: 35-41.

Bowles, R.T. and K.B. Beesley (1991) "Quality of Life, Migration to the Countryside and Rural Community Growth." In K.B. Beesley (ed.), *Rural and Urban Fringe Studies in Canada*. Atkinson College, York University, Geographical Monograph No. 21, 45-66.

Cape, E. (1987) "Aging Women in Rural Settings." In V.M. Marshall (ed.), *Aging in Canada: Social Perspectives*. Toronto: Fitzhenry and Whiteside, 84-99.

Coward, R.T. (1979) "Planning Community Services for the Rural Elderly: Implications from Research." *The Gerontologist* 19(3): 275-282.

Cronin, R.C., M.J. Drury and F.E. Gragg (1983) *An Evaluation of the FmHAAoA Demonstration Program of Congregate Housing in Rural Areas, Final Report*. Washington, D.C.: American Institute for Research.

Dahms, F.A. (1987) *Population Migration and the Elderly: Ontario 1971-1981*. Department of Geography, University of Guelph, Occasional Paper No. 9.

Feldman, E.J. (1981) *A Practical Guide to the Conduct of Field Research in the Social Sciences*. Boulder, Colorado: Westview Press.

Filion, P., A. Wister and E.J. Coblentz (1992) "Subjective Dimensions of Environmental Adaptation Among the Elderly: A Challenge to Models of Housing Policy." *Journal of Housing for the Elderly* 10(1/2): 3-32.

Forbes, W.F., J.A. Jackson and A.S. Kraus (1987) *Institutionalization of the Elderly in Canada*. Toronto: Butterworths.

Golant, S.M. (1991) "Matching Congregate Housing Settings with a Diverse Elderly Population: Research and Theoretical Considerations." *Journal of Housing for the Elderly* 9(1/2): 21-38.

Grant, P.R. and B. Rice (1983) "Transportation Problems of the Rural Elderly." *Canadian Journal on Aging* 2: 30-35.

Gutman, G. and N. Blackie (1984) *Innovations in Housing and Living Arrangements for Seniors*. Burnaby, B.C.: Gerontology Research Centre, Simon Fraser University.

Gutman, G. and G. Hodge (1990) *Housing and Support Service Needs and Preferences of Rural Seniors from Three Regions in Canada*. Burnaby, B.C.: Gerontology Research Centre, Simon Fraser University.

Health and Welfare Canada (1989) *Women in an Aging Society*. Report of Proceedings, National Workshop on Women in an Aging Society, Halifax, Nova Scotia, October 1988.

Hodge, G. (1984) *Shelter and Services for the Small-Town Elderly: The Role of Assisted Housing*. Ottawa: Canada Mortgage and Housing Corporation.

Hodge, G. (1987) "Assisted Housing for Ontario's Rural Elderly: Shortfalls in Product and Location." *Canadian Journal on Aging* 8(2): 141-154.

Hodge, G. (1991) *Seniors in Small Town British Columbia: Demographic Tendencies and Trends, 1961 to 1986*. Burnaby, B.C.: Gerontology Research Centre, Simon Fraser University.

Hodge, G. and M.A. Qadeer (1983) *Towns and Villages in Canada: The Importance of Being Unimportant.* Toronto: Butterworths.

Joseph, A.E. (1992) "On the Importance of Place in Studies of Rural Aging." *Journal of Rural Studies* 8(1): 111-119.

Joseph, A.E. and D. Cloutier (1991) "Elderly Migration and Its Implications for Service Provision in Rural Communities: An Ontario Perspective." *Journal of Rural Studies* 7(4): 433-444.

Joseph, A.E. and A.M. Fuller (1991) "Towards an Integrative Perspective on the Housing, Services and Transportation Implications of Rural Aging." *Canadian Journal on Aging* 10(2): 127-148.

Joseph, A.E. and A. Martin-Matthews (1993) "Growing Old in Aging Communities." *Journal of Canadian Studies* 28(1): 14-29.

Keating, N.C. (1991) *Aging in Rural Canada.* Toronto: Butterworths.

Kushman, J.E. and J. McClure (1985) *Tracking Changes in the Needs and Status of Older Americans.* University School of Rural Planning and Development/ Gerontology Research Centre, University of Guelph, Papers in Rural Aging No. 2.

Martin Matthews, A. (1988) "Variations in the Conceptualization and Measurement of Rurality." *Journal of Rural Studies* 4(2): 141-150.

Ministries of Health, Community and Social Services and Citizenship (1993) *Partnerships in Long-Term Care: A New Way to Plan, Manage and Deliver Services and Community Support–An Implementation Framework.* Toronto: Queen's Printer.

Monk, A. and L.W. Kaye (1991) "Congregate Housing for the Elderly: Its Need, Functions and Perspective." *Journal of Housing for the Elderly* 9(1/2): 5-19.

Nicholson, B. (1987) *Housing for Rural Small Town Seniors: Factors Influencing the Decision to Stay Living Independently.* University of Guelph, University School of Rural Planning and Development, unpublished M.A. thesis.

O'Bryant, S.L. (1983) "The Subjective Value of Home to Older Homeowners." *Journal of Housing for the Elderly* 1(1): 29-43.

Ontario Advisory Council on Senior Citizens (1992) *Rural Roots: Aging in Small and Rural Communities in Ontario.* Toronto: Queen's Printer.

Rosenberg, M.W., E.G. Moore and S.B. Ball (1989) "Components of Change in the Spatial Distribution of the Elderly Population in Ontario, 1976-1986." *The Canadian Geographer* 33(3): 218-229.

Scheidt, R.J. (1984) "A Taxonomy of Well-Being for Small-Town Elderly: A Case for Rural Diversity." *The Gerontologist* 24(1): 84-89.

Shimizu, K. (1988) "The Abbeyfield Model." In Gutman, G. and N. Blackie (eds.), *Housing the Very Old.* Burnaby, B.C.: Gerontology Research Centre, Simon Fraser University

Smit, B. and A.E. Joseph (1982) "Trade-Off Analysis of Preferences for Public Services." *Environment and Behavior* 14(2): 238-258.

Wister, A.V. (1989) "Privacy, Independence and Separateness in Living Arrangement Selection Among the Elderly: Research and Implications for Housing Policy." *Environments* 20(2): 26-35.

Chapter 8

Rural-Urban Differences
in Seniors' Neighbourhood Preferences

Zachary Zimmer
Neena Chappell

SUMMARY. Past research has indicated that it is important to consider the neighbourhood environment when addressing the issue of housing for seniors. Because rural and urban environments differ, neighbourhood preferences may vary as well. The following study attempts to ascertain the neighbourhood amenity preferences of a sample of rural and urban living elderly. A total of 1,408 seniors were asked to consider the importance of 11 amenities in a place to live. A factor analysis of the items indicates that planners need to consider three broad areas of amenities in a place to live: necessities, social interaction and life enrichment. Bivariate crosstabulations and multiple regression results demonstrate the importance of social in-

Zachary Zimmer, MA, is a Doctoral Candidate in the Population Studies Center and Department of Sociology, University of Michigan, and Research Associate at the Centre on Aging, University of Victoria. Neena Chappell, PhD, is Director of the Centre on Aging, University of Victoria, Victoria, British Columbia, Canada V8W 2Y2.

The data for this study was provided from the Canadian government's National Centres of Excellence program, funded by: the Medical Research Council; the National Health Research Development Program; the National Science and Engineering Research Council; National Centres of Excellence program; and the Social Science and Humanities Research Council of Canada.

[Haworth co-indexing entry note]: "Rural-Urban Differences in Seniors' Neighbourhood Preferences." Zimmer, Zachary, and Neena Chappell. Co-published simultaneously in *Journal of Housing for the Elderly* (The Haworth Press, Inc.) Vol. 12, No. 1/2, 1997, pp. 105-124; and: *Shelter and Service Issues for Aging Populations: International Perspectives* (ed: Leon A. Pastalan) The Haworth Press, Inc., 1997, pp. 105-124. Single or multiple copies of this article are available for a fee from The Haworth Document Delivery Service [1-800-342-9678, 9:00 a.m. - 5:00 p.m. (EST). E-mail address: getinfo@haworth.com].

teraction amenities to rural elders, confirming the instrumental importance that social relations serve for those living in rural areas. *[Article copies available for a fee from The Haworth Document Delivery Service: 1-800-342-9678. E-mail address: getinfo@haworth.com]*

INTRODUCTION

Rural living elderly differ in a number of important ways from their urban counterparts. There are differences in income and health status, as well as in the quality and quantity of social interaction. In addition, rural and urban neighbourhood environments tend to differ. Rural seniors are more isolated, hence transportation and accessibility to amenities becomes an issue. These differences suggest that the environmental needs of rural and urban seniors may differ.

A substantial amount of past research has explored the effect of the residential environment on housing and life satisfaction. This literature consistently states that the environment is an important determinant of satisfaction. However, very little of this research has examined differences between rural and urban living elderly despite obvious dissimilarities in their living environments. Furthermore, with exception of Carp and Carp (1982), seniors themselves are rarely asked what they personally prefer in a place to live. This study attempts to address the void in the literature by examining the types of amenities that seniors consider important in a place to live, comparing the environmental preferences of rural and urban elders.

REVIEW OF LITERATURE

Studies which look at seniors and their neighbourhoods seldom compare rural and urban living seniors, despite the fact that there are fundamental differences in their living environments. These differences ultimately influence the types of amenities and facilities that are needed by each group. Previous research has indicated that, in terms of subjective measures of well-being and life satisfaction, rural elders tend to score better than urbanites (Donnenwerth, Guy and Norvell, 1978; Hynson, 1975; Lee and Lassey, 1980; Liang and Warfel, 1983). This is so despite the fact that urban seniors tend to have more money than rural seniors both in the United States and in Canada (Lassey and Lassey, 1985; Shapiro and Roos, 1984), be in better health (Lee and Cassidy, 1985; Palmore, 1983; Youmans, 1967), and have better access to important amenities like a medical centre and convenient transportation (Blieszner et al., 1987; Lassey and Lassey, 1985).

One reason that rural elderly rate their life satisfaction higher than urban seniors may be because of the quantity and quality of their social interaction with others (Lee and Cassidy, 1985; Winch and Greer, 1968). There is some debate on whether the frequency of social interaction is greater among rural or urban elderly. While some studies indicate that social contact is more frequent in rural areas (Winch and Greer, 1968), others do not (Lee and Whitback, 1987; Strain and Chappell, 1980). But, despite disagreements in the quantity of interaction, there is little doubt that the nature of social interaction differs (Liang and Warfel, 1983). Rural seniors do seem to seek out relations with family and friends which serve more instrumental purposes than their urban counterparts (Lee and Cassidy, 1985). That is, rural relationships more often satisfy specific daily living functions rather than providing only emotional support. For this reason, social relations have a fundamentally different role to play in day-to-day living for rural elders.

In short, rural elders are different from their urban counterparts in a number of ways including accessibility to amenities and social interaction. Although urban neighbourhoods provide better accessibility to resources, increased and different social interaction may act as a substitute for rural seniors. This suggests that the environmental needs of rural and urban seniors also differ.

According to Donald L. Foley (1980), in his article entitled "The Sociology of Housing,"

> there is increasing recognition that 'housing' comprises much more than physical shelter and that it especially encompasses the broader residential setting . . . (H)ousing comprises a complex bundle of considerations, including privacy, location, environmental amenities, symbolic characteristics, and investment. (Foley, 1980; 457)

Previous research which examines what seniors consider to be important amenities in a place to live is sparse. However, research has looked at the living environment in terms of neighbourhood, residential and housing satisfaction. There is substantial literature which supports the notion that housing satisfaction is also a function of macro or environmental factors, in addition to physical housing characteristics.

The importance of the environment in residential satisfaction has been carefully examined by M. Powell Lawton and associates (Lawton, 1977, 1980, 1983; Lawton and Cohen, 1974; Lawton and Nahemow, 1979; Lawton, Nahemow and Yeh, 1980). Lawton and Nahemow (1979) showed that environmental factors predict housing satisfaction better than personal, sociodemographic indicators. For instance, increased age concentration of seniors positively effects activity participation levels, housing satisfaction and the number of friendships that seniors build with others in the area. Lawton, Nahemow and Yeh (1980) demonstrated that a series of dependent variables representing neighbourhood, residential and housing factors were significantly influenced by neighbourhood enriching facilities (like a church, movie theatre, restaurant, library, etc.), age segregation and a medical centre nearby. Lawton (1980) argues that housing satisfaction may be more a factor of environmental characteristics than either personal characteristics or the physical nature of the house itself. In addition, the closer the distance to resources which influence satisfaction, the greater the utilization of those resources.

Other research has determined that various macro and environmental factors influence older adults. For instance, the effect of age homogeneity (Lawton and Nahemow, 1979; Lawton, Nahemow and Yeh, 1980; Siegel, 1985), location and size of community (Leung, 1987; Rodgers, 1980), health factors (Barresi, Ferraro and Hobey, 1984; Windley and Scheidt, 1983), safety and aesthetic qualities (Jirovec, Jirovec and Bosse, 1984 and 1985) have all been shown to have an impact in promoting well-being and life and residential satisfaction.

In sum, past research which looks at the elderly and their neighbourhood environments supports the notions that accessibility of amenities can influence housing satisfaction. Hence, site location is important when planning housing for the elderly. A good location, containing the amenities which seniors consider to be important, can enhance their daily lives. Yet, only one study was found which asks seniors themselves about their preferences of nearby amenities.

Carp and Carp (1982) addressed this issue with a limited sample of seniors. In their study, 90 women, aged 60 and older, were asked about their preference for locating a variety of amenities within walking distance of their home. The attempt was to define the ideal residential area for seniors. Carp and Carp found that basic services and facilities rated highly. Among these, the highest ratings were given to a bus stop that takes you where you want to go, a favourite grocery store, their own bank, and a favourite drug store. In general, 17 basic service items were ranked higher than 12 life enrichment services and facilities. This study took place in Oakland, California, a large metropolitan centre, and did not compare rural and urban living seniors.

The present study goes further in the examination of seniors and their living environments by determining what seniors consider to be important amenities in a place to live, and examining the rural and urban differences in their responses. Considering the instrumental significance of social interaction for rural elderly, it may be hypothesized that socially related amenities would have greater importance for a rural population. However, because urbanites have better accessibility to a number of facilities, such as health services, it is also likely that rural living elderly have greater need in a number of these basic need areas.

DATA AND METHODS

The data utilized for these analyses come from the Canadian Aging Research Network needs assessment, a project which specifically aims at determining the needs of seniors in rural and urban areas throughout the Canadian province of Manitoba. Manitoba has one major metropolitan centre and communities outside of that centre are truly remote. That is, because of the low population density in Manitoba, not only are they far from the major city, they are generally far from other smaller communities as well. The notion of rurality can therefore be isolated with relative ease. Hence, this project, involving interviewing throughout the province of Manitoba, provides an ideal database for comparing rural versus urban elderly.

The needs assessment involved personal interviews lasting an average of 1 hour and 15 minutes. The total sample comprised 1,406 seniors, 65 years of age and older, living in Manitoba. One-half of the respondents were residents of Winnipeg, the only large urban centre in the province, while the other half of the sample was chosen from 8 smaller communities throughout the province, with populations ranging from about 2,000 to 10,000 inhabitants. For the purpose of this analysis, the Winnipeg respondents are coded as urban residents while the others are coded as rural residents.

The sampling design involved a two stage strategy. First, nine sites were selected from which the sample was drawn. Second, individuals from each site were chosen for personal interviews. The choice of sites was purposive, using the following criteria: an equal number of rural sites relatively near and far from the metropolitan centre were included, only sites with population sizes of about 2,000 inhabitants or more were selected, sites with a high proportion of elderly living in the community were considered, and an equal number of rural sites with and without the availability of a Provincial Department of Health office were included. Selection of respondents within sites used a random sample, stratified by age and sex, drawn from the list of medicare recipients in the designated sites. (The province provides universal medical coverage to its residents.) Potential respondents were first contacted by telephone at which time an appointment for the interview was arranged. Respondents were, in the vast majority of cases, interviewed in their own homes. The response rate for this study was 78%. A detailed description of the sample and methods of data collection can be found in Zimmer and Segall (1992).

As part of this project, seniors were asked about what amenities are important in a place to live by the following question: "We are interested in finding out what people consider to be important when looking for a place to live . . . For each item that I name, I would like to know if you consider it to be an important feature in a place to live." Respondents were then read a list of 11 amenities that could be located nearby. These were: a food store, a bank, a medical centre, a library, a pharmacy, a senior centre, a place to pay bills, a park, a post office, friends and relatives, and other seniors. A 3-point scale was utilized for the responses. Each amenity could be judged as being *very important* (scored 2), *slightly important* (scored 1), or *not important* (scored 0) in a place to live.

The 11 amenities were subjected to a principal component factor analysis in order to discover the underlying patterns in the data, whether the various amenities could be grouped into categories representing broader areas, and in order to simplify analyses. Based on the factored groupings, three indices were created from the 11 items which were later treated as dependent variables for multivariate analyses. The indices were created additively by summing the responses which combine to form each of the three factors. The resultant variables represent three broad areas of amenities: the importance of necessity amenities (bank, food store, pharmacy, place to pay bills, medical centre and post office), the importance of social interaction amenities (other seniors, friends and relatives and senior centre), and the importance of life enrichment amenities (library and park). Since responses for each amenity were coded as 0 (not important), 1 (slightly important) and 2 (very important), the first index, necessities, being derived from 6 items, has a possible low score of 0 and a high score of 12. Similarly, the social interaction index ranges in score from 0 to 6 and the life enrichment index ranges in score from 0 to 4. A test of reliability was conducted for each of the three indices. The necessity scale has an Alpha of .88 while the social interaction scale scores .63. The life enrichment index contains only 2 items.

The overall mean for the necessities index is 7.82. The social interaction index has an overall mean of 3.16 and the life enrichment index has an overall mean of 1.20. The average mean of the individual necessity items is 1.30. The social interaction items display an average mean of 1.05, while the average mean of the life enrichment items is .60. Hence, on average, the greatest importance is placed on the necessity items, followed by the social interaction items. The life enrichment items hold the least importance for the respondents.

In order to fully understand the relationship between the importance of amenities and place of residence, a number of controls are implemented which serve to isolate the effect of rurality. Previous research indicates that rural and urban populations can differ significantly in several areas: in terms of sociodemographic characteristics, health status characteristics, networking characteristics and residency characteristics. These characteristics could influence the wants and needs of seniors as far as important amenities in a place to live are concerned.

Important sociodemographic characteristics include the age, gender, marital status, education and income of the respondent. Age and education are measured in years on a continuous scale. Gender is dichotomous, while marital status is coded as a dummy variable indicating married or other. Income is measured on a 13-point scale of household income.

Rural and urban seniors also differ in terms of health status. The data set includes various indicators of health status, both objective and subjective. A measure for the number of chronic health conditions experienced by an individual is constructed by adding the number of affirmative responses to a list of 20 chronic conditions: heart trouble, stroke, high blood pressure, other circulation problems, kidney trouble, cancer, diabetes, breathing problems, palsy, thyroid trouble, stomach trouble, dental problems, emotional problems, foot or limb problems, skin trouble, arthritis, eye trouble, ear trouble, incontinence and other bladder problems. A measure for the number of health symptoms is constructed by adding the number of affirmative responses to a list of 11 symptomatic difficulties: dizziness, irregularity, tiredness, headaches, rashes, shortness of breath, pain, difficulty sleeping, loss of appetite, indigestion and depression. Whereas chronic conditions indicate the presence of an illness, symptoms indicate problems that are not necessarily specific to a condition but ones that might restrict the things that people do.

Respondents were also asked whether they experience 10 dexterity problems and 6 activities of daily living restrictions. The dexterity items include: opening medicine bottles, opening food boxes, opening milk cartons, wrapping food, opening plastic food containers, opening faucets, opening jars, peeling vegetables, using keys and turning doorknobs. The activities of daily living are: walking a city block, getting in and out of a car, getting in and out of the bathtub, getting in and out of bed, going up and down stairs and getting in and out of a chair. These two measures clearly indicate a level of mobility that could be important in determining the neighbourhood amenities preferred by seniors.

The final measure of health status is a subjective assessment of overall health. The single indicator used here is the one found in much gerontological research. Specifically, respondents were asked, "For your age, would you say in general your health is excellent, good, fair, poor or bad?" Seniors tend to report a relatively high level of self-assessed health status despite living with a number of chronic conditions, health symptoms, dexterity and activities of daily living restrictions. Seniors generally feel good about themselves and feel as if they cope well despite being faced with various health problems. It is for this reason that various measures of health are necessary in order to tap the range of health issues faced by seniors.

Some residency characteristics are important to consider in a study of this nature. These are characteristics which relate specifically to one's place of residence. Accessibility to resources is an important issue when looking at amenities preferred by seniors. Hence, a variable which looks at whether an individual already lives near the amenities in question has been included. This variable is constructed by adding the number of amenities referred to above that the respondent lives near. A separate variable for necessity, social interaction and life enrichment amenities is created.

Other important residency factors include a measure of mobility and ownership of housing. The number of years that an individual lives in a neighbourhood is an appropriate measure of mobility. Those who have more recently moved into a neighbourhood may have moved in order to be close to different amenities than those who have lived in the same neighbourhood for many years. Home ownership also may be an important determinant. Seniors who own as opposed to rent housing tend to have higher incomes, are younger, and are often in better health than renters. Many sell their homes when they get older and feel that it is difficult to maintain, or if they cannot afford to hire the help that they need to maintain the home. Renters, often living in seniors' housing, may therefore have specific needs in terms of amenities, which differ from owners. Ownership of housing is measured as a dichotomous variable indicating owned housing or other.

Finally, networking variables are important to consider. Those with a larger network of friends and family may put more emphasis on social interaction amenities and less on other types of facilities. For this reason, three networking variables are included: size of the overall network, household size, and whether an individual feels that they would like to have more contact with friends and family. Size of network is a continuous variable measured by adding the number of family and friends a respondent has, household size is continuous, and the contact variable is dichotomous indicating whether more contact is desired or not.

Table 1 displays the variables used as controls in the analysis of the importance of amenities in a place to live and, where necessary, the coding scheme utilized.

To explore the differences in rural versus urban responses to preferences of amenities, multiple regression analyses are used. This procedure allows for the simultaneous control of a number of variables while indi-

TABLE 1. Control Variables Used in the Analysis

Sociodemographic variables

— Age of respondent
— Gender of respondent (1 = Male; 0 = Female)
— Marital status (1 = Married; 0 = Other)
— Years of education
— Income (13-point household income scale)

Health status variables

— Self-assessed health status (5-point scale)
— Number of chronic health conditions (Ranging from 0 to 20)
— Number of health symptoms (Ranging from 0 to 11)
— Number of dexterity problems (Ranging from 0 to 10)
— Number of activities of daily living limitations (Ranging from 0 to 6)

Network variables

— Household size
— Size of network (Including friends and relatives)
— Wants more social contact with others (1 = Yes; 0 = No)

Residency variables

— Own housing (1 = Yes; 0 = No)
— Years lived in neighbourhood
— Lives near necessity, social interaction and life enrichment amenities (Coded as the number of amenities located nearby)
— Rural/urban residency (1 = Rural; 0 = Urban)

vidual effects are isolated. The regression equations which are discussed below have been tested for the assumptions of linearity and collinearity using the appropriate diagnostics.

RESULTS

First, the results of the factor analysis on the neighbourhood amenity items are discussed. The underlying patterns in the data are seen in Table 2. The first factor consists of those amenities which can be called *necessities*. In order of descending rotated factor scores, these necessities are: a bank nearby, a food store nearby, a pharmacy nearby, a place to pay bills nearby, a medical centre nearby, and a post office nearby. In total, this factor explains almost 42% of the variance with an eigenvalue of 4.6. The essence of the second factor is clear and includes those amenities which relate to *social interaction*. The items of this factor are: other seniors nearby, friends and relatives nearby and a senior centre nearby. Over 11% of the variance is explained by this factor which has an eigenvalue of 1.3. Finally, the third factor consists of two items which relate to *life enrichment*. These are: a library nearby and a park nearby. About 10% of the variance is explained by this factor which has an eigenvalue of 1.1.

None of the amenity items load highly onto more than one factor. The total variance explained is 63%. The three factors are clearly differentiated from one another and are theoretically suitable. The necessities factor includes important items for day-to-day living, such as shopping and health care. The social interaction factor includes items which are important for those who consider social relations to be vital to their life. The life enrichment factor includes items which, although not essential in day-to-day living, can increase life fulfillment.

Table 3 presents comparisons of the individual amenity items, and the mean scores for the three indices, for rural and urban respondents. Overall, necessity items were deemed to be very important more often than social interaction or life enrichment items. Nearly 60% rated having a food store nearby as being very important. This was the most highly rated item of the list of 11 amenities. Rural and urban residents were mixed in terms of the importance of necessity items. A higher proportion of rural residents stated that a pharmacy, a medical centre and a post office were very important features in a neighbourhood. Urban residents rated a bank, a food store and a place to pay bills as being more important than did rural residents. Despite mixed preference in terms of individual items, in total, rural respondents display a higher mean on the factor derived necessity index than urban residents (8.13 to 7.50). This difference of means is

TABLE 2. Principal Component Factor Analysis of Importance of Amenities*

FACTOR PATTERNS	1	2	3
1. <u>Necessities</u>			
– Bank nearby	.84		
– Food store nearby	.82		
– Pharmacy nearby	.78		
– Place to pay bills nearby	.75		
– Medical centre nearby	.70		
– Post office nearby	.67		
EIGENVALUE	4.6		
VARIANCE EXPLAINED	41.8%		
2. <u>Social Interaction</u>			
– Other seniors nearby		.81	
– Friends and relatives nearby		.73	
– Senior centre nearby		.60	
EIGENVALUE		1.3	
VARIANCE EXPLAINED		11.4%	
3. <u>Life Enrichment</u>			
– Library nearby			.78
– Park nearby			.75
EIGENVALUE			1.1
VARIANCE EXPLAINED			9.7%

<u>TOTAL VARIANCE EXPLAINED</u> = 62.9%

* Only rotated factor scores of .4 or over are reported.

significant at a .05 level. The larger mean score for rural respondents is, in part, due to the considerable differences in rating the importance of a medical centre. Fully, 65% of rural residents rated this amenity as very important compared to only 45% of urban respondents.

Although a high proportion of the total sample rated having friends and relatives nearby as very important (56.5%), a substantially lower proportion thought having other seniors (34.8%) or a senior centre (17%) nearby was a very important feature in a place to live. Rural residents consistently assessed these three social interaction amenities as more important than

TABLE 3. Percent Reporting Amenities Are Very Important, and Mean Index Scores, by Residency

	Rural residents (N = 704)	Urban residents (N = 704)	Total (N = 1406)
Necessities			
Bank nearby	45.1%	55.1%	50.1%
Food store nearby	54.0	65.2	59.6
Pharmacy nearby	51.7	47.9	49.8
Place to pay bills nearby	39.2	44.8	41.7
Medical centre nearby	65.3	45.3	55.3
Post office nearby	47.1	34.8	41.0
NECESSITY INDEX MEAN*	8.13	7.51	7.82
Social Interaction			
Other seniors nearby	39.9	29.7	34.8
Friends and relatives nearby	64.6	48.4	56.5
Senior centre nearby	19.0	15.1	17.0
SOCIAL INTERACTION INDEX MEAN*	3.53	2.79	3.16
Life Enrichment			
Library nearby	16.5	17.1	16.8
Park nearby	13.5	13.9	13.7
LIFE ENRICHMENT INDEX MEAN	1.23	1.17	1.20

* Difference of means significant at .05 level using a T-Test of significance.

did urban residents. For instance, 64.6% of rural respondents stated that having friends and relatives nearby was very important in a place to live, compared to 48.4% of urban residents. Rural elderly had a mean of 3.53 on the social interaction index compared to 2.79 for the urban elderly. This difference of means is significant at a .05 level. Hence, looking at individual items, or the total mean for the social interaction index, rural elderly consistently rate social interaction amenities as more important than their urban counterparts.

The two life enrichment items are, overall, rated much lower than most of the other items on the list. In contrast to the social interaction items, urban residents are the ones who more frequently stated that these amenities were very important features in a place to live. The differences here, however, are quite small. For instance, having a library nearby was assessed as being very important for 17.1% of urban respondents compared to 16.5% of ruralites. In fact, the rural group scores a slightly higher mean on the life enrichment index (1.23 to 1.17), though this difference is not significant.

Tables 4 through 6 display the results of three stepwise regression equations using the neighbourhood amenity indices as dependent variables in order to determine the effect of residency on the importance of necessities, social interaction and life enrichment amenities in general, controlling for other important correlates. Only those variables which statistically contribute to the models are displayed maintaining the greatest amount of parsimony in the equations.

Five variables are significant predictors of the necessity index. The number of necessities in one's neighbourhood is related to the importance placed on having these necessities nearby. Three of the demographic variables are significantly related to the necessity index. These are: income,

TABLE 4. Stepwise Regression Results

Dependent Variable = Necessity Index

Variable	Standardized Beta	T	Sig. of T	Change in r-SQ
# of necessity amenities already nearby	.20	7.56	.000	.036
Income	−.16	−5.29	.000	.029
Male gender	.14	4.07	.000	.016
# health symptoms	.11	3.82	.000	.011
Married	.10	3.28	.001	.008

R-Square = .10
F = 27.84
Sig. of F = .000

TABLE 5. Stepwise Regression Results

Dependent Variable = Social Interaction Index

Variable	Standardized Beta	T	Sig. of T	Change in r-SQ
# of social interaction amenities already nearby	.22	7.94	.000	.070
Income	−.11	−3.93	.000	.028
Rural residency	.12	4.12	.000	.016
Male gender	.11	3.99	.000	.014
# health symptoms	.09	3.16	.002	.008
Size of network	.09	3.14	.002	.006
Wants more contact	.07	2.42	.016	.004

R-Square = .15
F = 29.72
Sig. of F = .000

gender, and marital status. Those with lower income rated necessities more important than those with higher income; women rated having necessities nearby more important than men; and, married respondents rated nearby necessities as more important than non-married individuals. The health symptoms variable is also significant, with those reporting more symptoms placing more importance on having necessities nearby.

In the bivariate table, rural and urban residents had mixed responses to the importance of individual necessity amenities, though rural respondents scored higher on the overall index. When the other variables in the model are controlled for, rural-urban residency no longer significantly correlates with the necessity index. This suggests that the relationship that was found in the bivariate comparison of means is mediated by other factors which, when included in the model, explain the initial relationship. Rather, seniors who consider having necessities nearby tend more often to be married, women, those with lower income, in poorer health, and those who already live near these amenities, regardless of place of residency.

Moving on to the predictors of the social interaction index shown in

TABLE 6. Stepwise Regression Results

Dependent Variable = Life Enrichment Index

Variable	Standardized Beta	T	Sig. of T	Change in r-SQ
Education	.18	6.79	.000	.041
# of life enrichment amenities already nearby	.16	6.02	.000	.027

R-Square = .07
F   = 45.86
Sig. of F = .000

Table 5, the greater the number of social interaction amenities already available, again, the more important seniors rate these amenities to be. In addition, the greater the size of one's network, and the wish to have more contact with others, are also positively correlated with the importance that one places on social interaction amenities. Like the previous regression equation, income, gender and health symptoms are significant predictors. That is, lower income leads to feeling social interaction is more important, and women consider these amenities to be more important than men as do those with more symptomatic health problems.

Place of residency is a significant predictor of the importance of social interaction amenities. Those in rural areas consider living near other seniors, near friends and relatives and near a senior centre as being important in a neighbourhood.

The third regression equation considers the life enrichment index as the dependent variable, the results of which can be seen in Table 6. Only two significant variables emerge. Education contributes most to believing life enrichment amenities are important and having life enrichment amenities nearby is, once again, a significant predictor. Place of residency is not significantly related to the importance that older individuals place on nearby life enrichment amenities.

DISCUSSION

When addressing the subject of housing for seniors, it is important to consider more than just the built environment, but the neighbourhood surroundings as well. A good housing location, which allows for access to important amenities, is related to overall satisfaction for seniors. Differences between rural and urban living elderly and the environments in which they live suggest that their neighbourhood needs may differ. The present study attempted to fill a void in past research by contrasting the amenity preferences of seniors living in rural and urban areas in order to determine what seniors living in these areas consider to be important amenities in a place to live. By ascertaining the amenities that seniors themselves report as being very important, the results of this research have important implications for both researchers and planners of housing for seniors.

Overall, the above analysis has suggested which types of amenities are most important to seniors. Looking at the individual items, seniors rated having a food store nearby, having friends and relatives nearby, having a medical centre nearby and having a bank nearby as the most important amenities. At least 50% of the total sample rated these items as very important in a place to live. Besides having friends and relatives nearby, the other most highly rated items deal with necessities of life and taking care of daily business. Therefore, when choosing the most important amenities in a place to live, seniors choose those which serve a specific and necessary function.

When examining amenities in a place to live, it is clear that planners need to consider three differentiated categories. These are: those amenities which can be deemed as necessities, such as a food store; those which are important for social interaction, such as having other seniors nearby; and those which are life enrichment amenities, such as having a library in the neighbourhood.

A bivariate crosstabulation of the individual items that make up these broad categories showed that the social interaction items are consistently rated as being very important more often by rural elderly than by their urban counterparts. That is, a substantially higher percentage of rural elders reported that having other seniors, friends and relatives and a senior centre nearby is very important in a place to live. For instance, 65% of rural respondents rated having friends and relatives nearby as very important compared to only 48% for urban elderly. For the ruralites, this is the second highest rated item of the 11 amenities referred to. On the other hand, urban residents rated the life enrichment items as very important more frequently, although the differences found here are quite small. Finally, some necessity items are more important to one group and some to the other. For the rural group, the two health-related items, a medical centre and a pharmacy, are rated very important more often than they are for urban respondents, as is having a post office nearby. Conversely, urban respondents rated a food store, a place to pay bills and a bank as very important more often than urbanites. The medical centre item is rated higher by the rural group by a substantial margin. Fully, 65% of rural elderly rated a medical centre as very important compared to only 45% or urbanites. For this reason, the overall necessity index is higher for the rural residents. This finding also takes on some additional significance in light of previous research quoted above which shows ruralites to be disadvantaged in terms of access to medical services.

Overall, life enrichment amenities were given lower preference than necessities and social interaction amenities, while the necessity items are rated very important in a place to live most often. This confirms the results found by Carp and Carp (1982) in their study of a small group of urban elderly.

When other correlates are controlled for in a multivariate regression, the importance of social interaction among rural elderly is confirmed. However, the overall conclusion is clear: place of residence makes a difference only in terms of social interaction amenities. Nearby necessity and life enrichment amenities are equally important to seniors living in rural and urban areas. Instead of place of residence, the importance placed on necessities is related to the gender, marital status and income of the respondent, as well as the number of health symptoms that an individual experiences and the existence of necessities in the area already. The importance of life enrichment amenities relates to education and the existence of these amenities in the area already.

This conclusion makes sense in light of previous literature. In particular, since social interaction takes on a more instrumental role for seniors living in rural areas, it is reasonable that they would rate social interaction items as more important than do urban seniors. Transportation is one example of how rural elderly may utilize social relations for instrumental purposes. A study conducted by The Senior Citizens' Provincial Council in Saskatchewan (1982) estimated that those living on farms must drive an average of 16 miles to get to the doctor compared to 1 mile in the comparative urban area. Hence, urban residents not only have more facilities to choose from, they live nearer to them than do rural residents. For those who do not drive, public transportation is more readily accessible for urban elderly. Rural elderly, on the other hand, more often rely on others for transportation. These instrumental roles that relations take on makes social interaction amenities essential for rural elderly.

One interesting finding is that, in regards to all three broad amenity areas, those who already live near these facilities tend to rate them as being important amenities to have in the neighbourhood. This consistency needs to be addressed. There are two possible explanations. First, it is possible that seniors tend to move into neighbourhoods that already contain the amenities that they feel are important. This would involve a conscious decision on the part of the older adult at the time of moving to seek out the neighbourhood that suits their needs. Alternatively, if an individual has access to some facility, they will utilize it and perhaps gain an appreciation of its importance. In the end, an individual will tend to rate that amenity as being important to have in a neighbourhood. In other words, the greater the access and utilization of a facility, the more important having that facility becomes in the eyes of the user. Further study, utilizing longitudinal data, is clearly necessary in order to sort out which of these two explanations suit.

A lack of a significant result in terms of the effect of residency on the importance of life enrichment amenities is curious. It should be noted that explained variance in this equation was considerably low. The insignificant finding may be due to a weakness in the data rather than the actual similarity in preference found. That is, life enrichment facilities include more than just a park and a library, the only two items available in the data set. Urban residents have more and better access to theatres, restaurants and movie houses as well. Had these items been included, it is quite possible that urban seniors would have scored, on average, higher in terms of the life enrichment index than rural residents. The emergence of this dimension as conceptually distinct warrants further study in future research.

Although the neighbourhood environment exerts a great influence on the elderly, they are rarely consulted about what type of environment they prefer. This paper has demonstrated the utility in asking elderly about what they consider to be important amenities to have in their own neighbourhoods. Seniors tend to choose necessities over life enrichment facilities with some individual item differences based on rural and urban residency. Clearly, rural seniors choose social interaction amenities more frequently than urbanites, confirming the instrumental importance that social relations serve for those living in rural areas.

REFERENCES

Barresi Charles M., Kenneth F. Ferraro and Linda L. Hobey. 1984. "Environmental Satisfaction, Sociability, and Well-Being Among Urban Elderly." *International Journal of Aging and Human Development.* 18(4):277-293.
Blieszner Rosemary, William J. McAuley, Janette K. Newhouse and Jay A. Man-

cini. 1987. "Rural-Urban Differences in Service Use by Older Adults." Pp. 162-174 in *Aging, Health and Family: Long-Term Care*, edited by Timothy H. Brubaker. Beverly Hills, CA: Sage Publications.

Carp Frances M. and Abraham Carp. 1982. "The Ideal Residential Area." *Research on Aging*. 4(4):411-439.

Donnenwerth Gregory V., Rebecca F. Guy and Melissa J. Norvell. 1978. "Life Satisfaction Among Older Persons: Rural-Urban and Racial Comparisons." *Social Science Quarterly*. 59(3):578-583.

Foley Donald L. 1980. "The Sociology of Housing." *Annual Review of Sociology*. 6:457-478.

Hynson Lawrence M., Jr. 1975. "Rural-Urban Differences in Satisfaction Among the Elderly." *Rural Sociology*. 40(1):64-66.

Jirovec Ronald L., Mary Marmoll Jirovec and Raymond Bosse. 1985. "Residential Satisfaction as a Function of Micro and Macro Environmental Conditions Among Urban Elderly Men." *Research on Aging*. 7(4):601-616.

Jirovec Ronald L., Mary Marmoll Jirovec and Raymond Bosse. 1984. "Environmental Determinants of Neighborhood Satisfaction Among Urban Elderly Men." *The Gerontologist*. 24(3):261-265.

Lassey William R. and Marie L. Lassey. 1985. "The Physical Health Status of the Rural Elderly." Pp. 79-104 in *The Elderly in Rural Society*, edited by Raymond T. Coward and Gary R. Lee. New York: Springer Publishing.

Lawton M. Powell. 1983. "Environment and Other Determinants of Well-Being in Older People." *The Gerontologist*. 23(4):349-357.

Lawton M. Powell. 1980. *Environment and Aging*. Monterey, CA: Brooks/Cole Publishing Company.

Lawton M. Powell. 1977. "Environments for Older Persons." *The Humanist*. 37(5):20-24.

Lawton M. Powell and Jacob Cohen. 1974. "Environment and the Well-Being of Elderly Inner-City Residents." *Environment and Behavior*. 6(2):194-211.

Lawton M. Powell and Lucille Nahemow. 1979. "Social Areas and the Wellbeing of Tenants in Housing for the Elderly." *Multivariate Behavioral Research*. 14(4):463-484.

Lawton M. Powell, Lucille Nahemow and Tsong-Min-Yeh. 1980. "Neighborhood Environment and the Wellbeing of Older Tenants in Planned Housing." *International Journal of Aging and Human Development*. 11(3):211-227.

Lee Gary R. and Margaret L. Cassidy. 1985. "Family and Kin Relations of the Rural Elderly." Pp. 151-192 in *The Elderly in Rural Society*, edited by Raymond T. Coward and Gary R. Lee. New York: Springer Publishing.

Lee Gary R. and Marie L. Lassey. 1980. "Rural-Urban Differences Among the Elderly: Economic, Social and Subjective Factors." *Journal of Social Issues*. 36(2):62-74.

Lee Gary R. and Les B. Whitback. 1987. "Residential Location and Social Relations Among Older Persons." *Rural Sociology*. 52(1):89-97.

Leung Hok Lin. 1987. "Housing Concerns of Elderly Homeowners." *Journal of Aging Studies*. 1(4):379-391.

Liang Jersey and Becky L. Warfel. 1983. "Urbanism and Life Satisfaction Among the Aged." *Journal of Gerontology.* 38(1):97-106.

Palmore Erdman. 1983. "Health Care Needs of the Rural Elderly." *International Journal of Aging and Human Development.* 18(1):39-45.

Rodgers Willard. 1980. "Residential Satisfaction in Relation to Size of Place." *Social Psychology Quarterly.* 43(4):436-441.

Senior Citizens' Provincial Council (Saskatchewan). 1982. "A Survey of the Transportation Needs of the Rural Elderly."

Shapiro Evelyn and Leslie L. Roos. 1984. "Using Health Care: Rural/Urban Differences Among the Manitoba Elderly." *The Gerontologist.* 24(3):270-274.

Siegel David I. 1985. "Homogeneous versus Heterogeneous Areas for the Elderly." *Social Service Review.* 59(2):216-238.

Strain Laurel A. and Neena L. Chappell. 1980. "Rural-Urban Differences Among Adult Day Care Participants in Manitoba." *Canadian Journal on Aging.* 2(4):197-209.

Winch Robert F. and Scott A. Greer. 1968. "Urbanism, Ethnicity and Extended Families." *Journal of Marriage and the Family.* 30(1):40-45.

Windley Paul G. and Rick J. Scheidt. 1983. "Housing Satisfaction Among Rural Small-Town Elderly: A Predictive Model." *Journal for Housing for the Elderly.* 1(2):57-68.

Youmans E. Grant. 1967. "Health Orientations of Older Rural and Urban Men." *Geriatrics.* 22(10):139-147.

Zimmer Zachary and Alexander Segall. 1992. "Needs Assessment Survey Methodology." Technical report written for the Canadian Aging Research Network. Centre on Aging, University of Manitoba.

Chapter 9

Aging and the Demographic Ecology of Urban Areas

Elia Werczberger

SUMMARY. This paper examines effects of demographic aging on the urban ecology, in particular, on the spatial concentration of the elderly. It uses a quasi-dynamic simulation model based on a simple accounting framework to analyze the combined effects of the aging of households and of residential buildings. Three factors are shown to bring about the spatial integration of different age groups: spatial mobility, nondurable housing and household dissolution. Hypothetical examples serve to demonstrate the effect of changing the parameters affecting these processes. If all households have the same preferences for proximity to the center, constant population size results in a completely integrated age distribution. In a growing city, new households concentrate at the periphery, creating a gradually outward moving suburban ring of young households. As these neighborhoods become older, an integrated age distribution develops. On the other hand, age-specific preferences regarding the demographic composition of neighborhoods and relocation lead to a lasting spatial concentration of elderly households. *[Article copies available for a fee from The Haworth Document Delivery Service: 1-800-342-9678. E-mail address: getinfo@haworth.com]*

Elia Werczberger, PhD, is affiliated with The Public Policy Program, Tel-Aviv University, Tel-Aviv 69978, Israel.

[Haworth co-indexing entry note]: "Aging and the Demographic Ecology of Urban Areas." Werczberger, Elia. Co-published simultaneously in *Journal of Housing for the Elderly* (The Haworth Press, Inc.) Vol. 12, No. 1/2, 1997, pp. 125-145; and: *Shelter and Service Issues for Aging Populations: International Perspectives* (ed: Leon A. Pastalan) The Haworth Press, Inc., 1997, pp. 125-145. Single or multiple copies of this article are available for a fee from The Haworth Document Delivery Service [1-800-342-9678, 9:00 a.m. - 5:00 p.m. (EST). E-mail address: getinfo@haworth.com].

INTRODUCTION

The Problem

One of the striking demographic characteristics of industrial and post-industrial societies is the continuing decline in mortality and fertility. As its consequence, the elderly in developed nations are becoming a steadily growing proportion of the population. Moreover, they tend to concentrate, usually in older neighborhoods located close to the center of the city (Newcomer, 1986; Pampel and Choldin, 1978; Smith and Hiltner, 1975). Both processes, the aging of the population and the spatial clustering of the elderly, have significant implications for the urban ecology and affect many aspects of urban development and public policy. In particular, they are likely to have important effects on social programs which focus on the adult population (see, e.g., Huttman and Gurewitsch, 1987; and others). It would therefore indeed be valuable to know, whether spatial concentrations of the elderly are a temporary phenomenon, and which factors may affect their future development.

This paper presents and applies a simple simulation model of structural and demographic aging to the study of the urban spatial structure. Its purpose is to clarify the role of a number of factors hypothesized to affect the demographic ecology: population growth, age-specific differences in mobility, household dissolution, and the withdrawal of older dwellings from the housing market through demolition. However, the model ignores economic factors such as income, housing quality and access to work or services, which are most effectively dealt with by standard economic models of the housing market. The specific purpose of this paper is to clarify the effect of mobility and structural aging on the demographic ecology; the complexity of a full economic housing market model did not seem to be justified by the additional realism gained.

Background: Demographic Factors

The spatial distribution of the elderly is usually explained by two sets of factors affecting their housing demand: reduced spatial mobility and age-related preferences for dwelling type and location. Both may contribute to the concentration of the aged in older housing and older neighborhoods.

The process of spatial differentiation by age is, however, more complex. New households are constantly being formed, are aging, and dissolve because of divorce, illness and death. They typically move several times during their lifetime in response to changes in income, housing needs and work location. With increasing age, however, the financial and psychological costs of relocation become higher and the propensity to change residence diminishes (Spear and Meyer, 1988; Lawton and Kleban, 1973). The elderly thus tend to "age in place" or to move over short distances only. Reasons for relocation cited include, in particular, reduced demand for space, the desire for proximity to relatives and excessive housing costs. If the elderly move, they are inclined to choose older housing units, because of their location or lower price and not to move over great distances (Golant, 1975; Wiseman, 1986; Rogers, 1989). On the other hand, regarding interregional migration, there is also some evidence to the contrary. Retirement migration to rural areas seems to play a significant role in the process of counterurbanization in Great Britain and in Germany (Champion, 1989). In the United States, it is the retirement migration of elderly persons to Florida which seems to contrast with the stereotype of the immobile elderly.

Locational preferences of elderly households are related also to problems and difficulties associated with age (Wiseman, 1986). Deteriorating health and declining income reduce daily mobility and thus increase the importance of access to specialized services and facilities (Huttman, 1986; Wiseman, 1986). Together with the smaller household size of the retired population, these factors also reduce demand for low density housing because of its high costs of operation, maintenance, and taxes. Older people have therefore been observed to concentrate in centrally located and densely developed neighborhoods, where they are more likely to find housing appropriate for their needs and neighbors with similar preferences and life styles (Smith and Hiltner, 1975). On the other hand, many elderly prefer proximity to their social network of friends of similar age and are therefore reluctant to leave their neighborhood (Ginsberg, 1988).

Structural Deterioration

Interacting with the effects of demographic aging and of the relocation of residents, there is a second set of processes: the deterioration of buildings and houses with age. Housing maintenance and the cost of modernization become over time increasingly expensive, until demolition remains the most efficient policy. The result is physical decline and economic obsolescence of housing, which in homogeneous areas may lead to the neighborhood life-cycle described, e.g., by Downs (1981).

Most recent research on the life cycle of neighborhoods is based on the theoretical framework of filtering, i.e., the decline in value of residential buildings and the replacement of the population by households of lower income (see, e.g., Lowry, 1960; Grigsby, 1987; and Baer and Williamson,

1986, for a comprehensive survey). The model presumes the existence of separate housing submarkets, which differ with regard to the quality and value of buildings and the income of the residents. Filtering is conceptualized as the change in the relative quality or value of housing or in population composition associated with the shift of a neighborhood to a different submarket (Grigsby, 1987). The transition is explained as the consequence of spatial externalities or of the physical deterioration of the housing stock (Brueckner, 1977). Human aging enters the model only indirectly through its correlate, the decrease in income after retirement and its impact on the demand for housing services.

Demolition of dwellings forces households to move, regardless of their preferences for relocation. The actual effect on the urban demographic ecology depends on the existing spatial distribution of the different age groups and on the location preferences of the involuntary movers. If the population living in older buildings is homogeneous, demolition should result in demographic integration. If the age of the inhabitants is highly heterogeneous, no effect may result.

A MODEL OF URBAN GROWTH AND AGING HOUSING

Conceptual Structure and Assumptions

Appendix A introduces a simulation model based on a quasi-dynamic accounting framework of the housing market. To keep the presentation accessible also to the reader who is not mathematically inclined, the discussion in this section concentrates on the central assumptions and the conceptual framework. The details of the analytical structure are relegated to the appendix.

We begin by introducing a few assumptions necessary to keep the model structure transparent and relatively simple. First of all, we assume total demand and supply for housing to be exogenous. In addition, the population is taken to be differentiated only by age, but homogeneous with respect to socioeconomic characteristics such as income. Age-specific preferences with regard to housing and location are also disregarded.

The housing market is equally simplified. Dwellings are presumed to be homogeneous, except for age and location, yet quality is taken to remain constant. The cost of upkeep, however, increases with the age of the structure, until further maintenance ceases to be profitable and the unit is demolished. Dwellings thus differ only with regard to two characteristics, age and location (zone, neighborhood), with regard to which households are taken to be indifferent.[1]

Two central factors affecting the urban ecology are therefore ignored: differences in socioeconomic status and income and discrepancies in housing characteristics, such as quality, size, type of structure, and quality of neighborhood.[2] The likelihood that a household is assigned to a dwelling unit is consequently independent of its income, the price of the unit or its location in the urban area. The effect of age-dependent differences in preferences is modeled using a stochastic utility framework imbedded in a simplified version of the Lowry model.

The Algorithm

Given any allocation of households to dwellings, the model calculates the allocation in the next period in four stages: (1) First, it provides an estimate of the demand for vacant dwellings based on the number of newly formed and moving households. (2) Next, it determines the supply of vacant dwellings by zone, based on the number of units vacated and demolished. (3) Where applicable, age specific location preferences are determined. (4) The fourth stage simulates the allocation of movers to vacant dwellings.

The driving forces for changes in the demographic ecology are hypothesized to be four: household mobility, the aging of households, their dissolution, and the demolition of residential structures.

Evaluation of the Model

Using the simulation model described in Appendix A, the next section examines the dynamic changes in the demographic ecology of an urban area. It does so by simulating the effect of changing each of the parameters hypothesized to affect the spatial distribution of the elderly. The analysis begins by assuming a constant, but immobile population and durable housing. It then considers the effect of relaxing each of these restrictive assumptions. The demographic distribution of the elderly will be shown to be a function of three factors: the rate of survival of households, their mobility, and the rate of demolition of buildings.[3] The last two paragraphs consider the effect of a growing population and of locational preferences regarding the demographic composition of the residential areas.

The simulations are performed for a monocentric city located in a featureless plane. All employment and shopping are assumed to take place in the CBD (central business district), which is situated on the coast of the ocean, but is so small that its spatial extent can be ignored (see Figure 1).

FIGURE 1. Stable Population and Durable Housing: Changing Initial Allocation

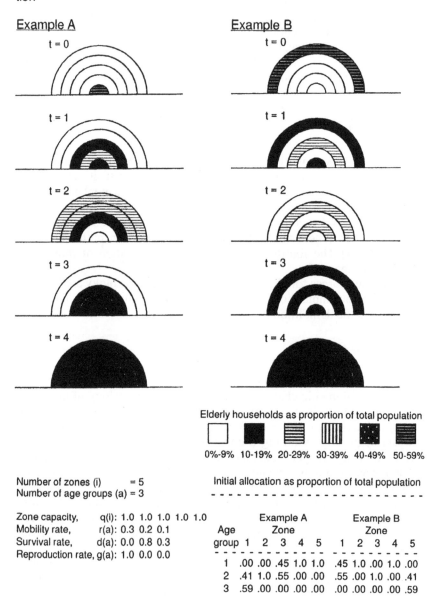

Number of zones (i)   = 5
Number of age groups (a) = 3

Initial allocation as proportion of total population

Zone capacity,	q(i): 1.0 1.0 1.0 1.0 1.0
Mobility rate,	r(a): 0.3 0.2 0.1
Survival rate,	d(a): 0.0 0.8 0.3
Reproduction rate,	g(a): 1.0 0.0 0.0

Age group	Example A Zone 1	2	3	4	5	Example B Zone 1	2	3	4	5
1	.00	.00	.45	1.0	1.0	.45	1.0	.00	1.0	.00
2	.41	1.0	.55	.00	.00	.55	.00	1.0	.00	.41
3	.59	.00	.00	.00	.00	.00	.00	.00	.00	.59

By letting access to the center be equal from every direction, the boundary of the urban area can be approximated by a half-circle. To examine dynamic changes in the spatial pattern, the area is divided into a set of concentric half-rings of equal width, which are taken to be homogeneous except for their distance from the center. If the population is in equilibrium, there must be a feature which compensates households living farther away. Following the usual assumptions made in urban economics, we assume that households trade off distance for space. The residential density in each of the concentric rings can then be assumed to decline with increasing distance from the center, so that each ring has the same capacity for residential development. This does not affect the generality of the results, but simplifies their presentation.

Note that the parameters used in the simulation are not intended to reflect real life conditions, but rather to facilitate the graphic display of the results. Using realistic parameters would not have changed the conclusions, but would have made their presentation much more difficult.

THE SPATIAL DISTRIBUTION OF THE ELDERLY

No Spatial Mobility

Four simplifying assumptions are introduced as benchmark. Their implications can be obtained by a simple thought experiment. Assume constant population size and perfectly durable housing. Furthermore, suppose that all households have the same life span and are spatially immobile, so that they do not relocate until dissolution. Given these conditions, it is easy to see that the degree of segregation must remain constant, as dissolving households are immediately replaced by newly formed ones. Consequently, if the initial age distribution is segregated, it will remain so forever, and if it is integrated, it will stay so as well. However, the location of age clusters will change when concentrations of older households are replaced by younger ones.

Assume next that the life span of households varies between age groups, but that once a household has been assigned to a dwelling, it does not relocate until dissolution. Only newly formed households move then into vacant dwellings, replacing households of any other age group and thus increasing age heterogeneity in that neighborhood. Variance in life expectancy thus leads to the spatial integration of different age groups.

Figure 1 shows for two arbitrary initial allocations, how an originally age-segregated spatial pattern with durable housing develops within a few periods into a completely integrated pattern. Since we assumed that the demographic composition does not affect the spatial choice of relocating households, the initial spatial pattern has no effect on the rate of demographic integration.

The Effect of Spatial Mobility and Non-Durable Housing

The relocation of households also accelerates demographic integration. It has thus the same desegregating effect as household dissolution, because households are assumed not to differ by age with regard to the factors which affect their choice of a neighborhood. The integrating influence of household mobility can be demonstrated by varying relocation rates (Figure 2). Note that the higher the mobility rate is, the faster the age distribution becomes homogeneous.

If the cost of maintaining residential structures is increasing with the age of the building, demolition becomes necessary because of excessively expensive maintenance. It forces households living in older buildings to relocate, and thus, also accelerates age integration, as more young households move into the new structures than had been living in the demolished ones. The graphic illustration of this example was omitted, since the integrating effect of increasing demolition rates is exactly analogous to the effect of higher mobility rates.

If, however, housing quality deteriorates with age, quality preferences will have to be introduced. These are likely to be a function of income and thus of the age of the household. The elderly and the very young tend to have a lower income compared with the rest of the population. We would thus expect these two groups to concentrate in older, less expensive and more centrally located housing. A satisfactory analysis of this issue would require modelling location choice by explicitly considering differences in income and endogenous prices, which is not feasible with the present approach.

Growing Population

Consider next a monocentric city with nondurable housing, whose population increases as a result of natural growth. Suppose also that commuting costs are non-negligible. Given our assumptions regarding the homogeneity of housing quality, the city will remain compact without leapfrogging. New construction then takes place at the periphery of the built-up area, forming a "ring" of new neighborhoods with a predominantly young population. When these households age in place, the proportion

FIGURE 2. Stable Population and Durable Housing: Changing Mobility Rates

Example A: Low mobility

Mobility rate: m(a) 0.3 0.2 0.1

Example B: High mobility

Mobility rate: m(a) 0.8 0.4 0.2

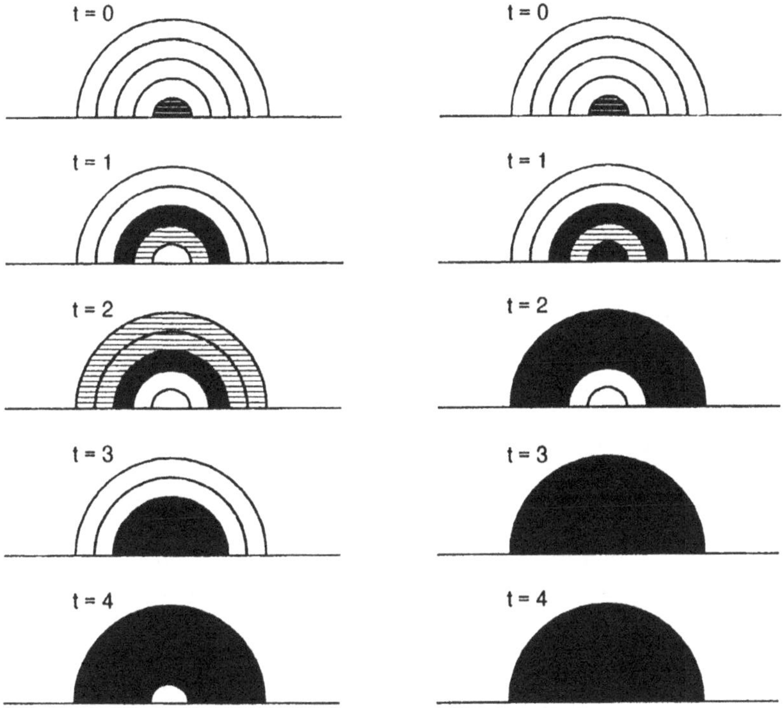

Elderly households as proportion of total population

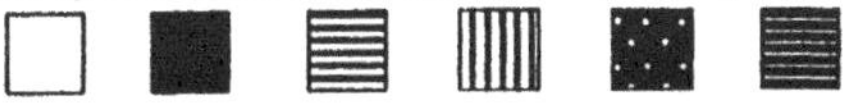

| 0%-9% | 10-19% | 20-29% | 30-39% | 40-49% | 50-59% |

Number of zones (i)   = 5
Number of age groups (a) = 3

Zone capacity,   q(i): 1.0 1.0 1.0 1.0 1.0
Survival rate,   d(a): 0.2 0.1 0.05
Reproduction rate, g(a): 1.0 0.0 0.0

Initial allocation as proportion of total population
- -

Example A

Age group	Zone 1	2	3	4	5
1	.00	.00	.45	1.0	1.0
2	.41	1.0	.55	.00	.00
3	.59	.00	.00	.00	.00

of elderly rises. However, because of mobility and mortality, the demographic composition becomes even in these areas more heterogeneous with the passing of time. After the first cohort of households has been replaced, an integrated pattern will begin to develop.

Figure 3 presents an example for this kind of development, assuming that growth is limited to a few (here six) periods. Note the outward shift of the "ring" of elderly households in periods 2, 3 and 4. These concentrations are formed in relatively homogeneous neighborhoods inhabited by young households that age in place. When these dissolve, they are replaced by younger households, some of which again age in place. In the example shown in Figure 3, the proportion of elderly in the center thus grows again in the fifth period, though at a lower rate because of the integration due to spatial mobility. If household mobility is low, the age distribution in each neighborhood may go through several decaying cycles. Fluctuations may continue for some time, even after growth has come to a halt, because of the effect of migration on demographic segregation. After growth ceases, the age distribution becomes within few periods completely integrated.

Preferences Regarding Neighborhood Composition

In the preceding sections, households were assumed to be indifferent to the social composition of the neighborhood and the distance of the move. Explicit consideration of location preferences does, of course, affect the spatial distribution of the elderly. Suppose that locational preferences are a function of the demographic composition of the neighborhood, such as when the elderly prefer areas with high concentrations of adult households. If for any exogenous reason, such as the sudden influx of a homogeneous population, a spatial concentration of the elderly is created, it will persist for some time. In the extreme case, the clustering of the elderly will continue until the old buildings are demolished and replaced by new construction. At that point the remaining elderly are forced to relocate. When new buildings are constructed on the site, no clusters of elderly will remain which would be more attractive to older households than to younger ones. Figure 4 shows how preference for proximity to concentrations of the elderly results in the development of an elderly ghetto in the center, instead of the expected greying of the suburbs. This concentration of elderly may occur when a homogeneous but immobile group of younger households ages in place.

If moving older households prefer to stay within the same neighborhood, the integrative effect of mobility is reduced. Existing concentrations of adult households that age in place are then also likely to persist. The

FIGURE 3. Growing Population and Non-Durable Housing

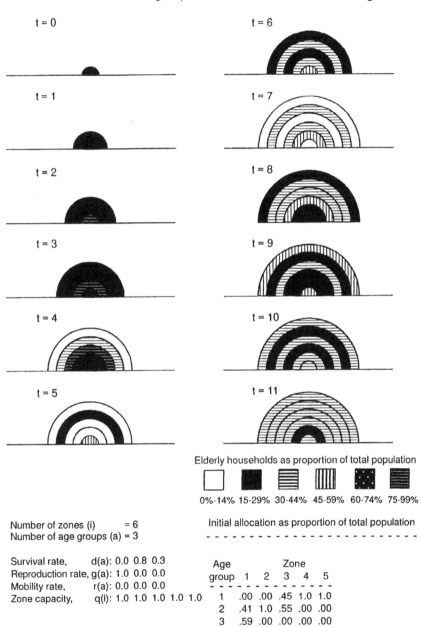

Elderly households as proportion of total population

0%-14% 15-29% 30-44% 45-59% 60-74% 75-99%

Number of zones (i)   = 6
Number of age groups (a) = 3

Initial allocation as proportion of total population

Survival rate,   d(a): 0.0 0.8 0.3
Reproduction rate, g(a): 1.0 0.0 0.0
Mobility rate,   r(a): 0.0 0.0 0.0
Zone capacity,   q(i): 1.0 1.0 1.0 1.0 1.0

Age group	Zone 1	2	3	4	5
1	.00	.00	.45	1.0	1.0
2	.41	1.0	.55	.00	.00
3	.59	.00	.00	.00	.00

FIGURE 4. Externalities with a Growing Population and Non-Durable Housing

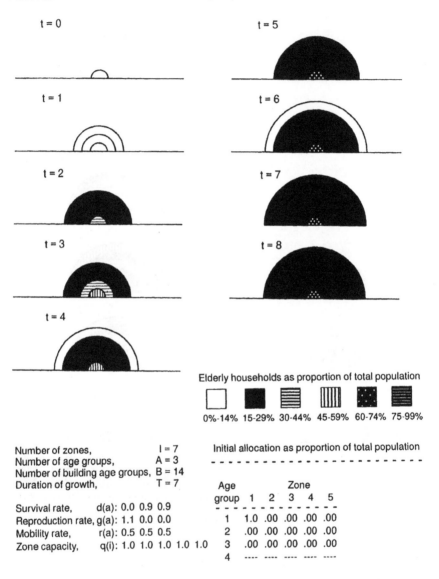

Elderly households as proportion of total population

0%-14%   15-29%   30-44%   45-59%   60-74%   75-99%

Number of zones,	$I = 7$	
Number of age groups,	$A = 3$	
Number of building age groups,	$B = 14$	
Duration of growth,	$T = 7$	

Survival rate, $d(a)$: 0.0 0.9 0.9
Reproduction rate, $g(a)$: 1.1 0.0 0.0
Mobility rate, $r(a)$: 0.5 0.5 0.5
Zone capacity, $q(i)$: 1.0 1.0 1.0 1.0 1.0

Initial allocation as proportion of total population

Age group	Zone 1	2	3	4	5
1	1.0	.00	.00	.00	.00
2	.00	.00	.00	.00	.00
3	.00	.00	.00	.00	.00
4	----	----	----	----	----

effect in terms of demographic segregation is the same as the consequences to be expected from low spatial mobility of the elderly.

DISCUSSION AND CONCLUSION

In this essay, a number of factors have been shown to affect the demographic ecology of urban areas. Some lead to the spatial integration of the elderly and some to their segregation.

Aging generally reduces the spatial mobility of households and increases their mortality. Ceteris paribus, both effects tend to support the spatial integration of different age groups. So does structural aging, which results in the demolition of old buildings and neighborhoods and forces the relocation of households, which otherwise would have stayed put.

The spatial clustering of older households, on the other hand, may be the result of two quite different processes. In a growing city, such concentrations are created when young households move into new neighborhoods and age in place, as suggested by the notion of the "greying" of the suburbs. It may also result from locational preferences of elderly movers, which seek proximity to households of their own age or buildings and neighborhoods suited to their needs. Such processes are likely to extend the existence of grey ghettoes longer than would be expected, if they were just the result of aging in place.

This paper ignored the third, and perhaps most important, factor contributing to the creation of elderly concentrations: the market and the role of income, housing quality, and prices. Similar to locational preferences and externalities, they seem to promote age segregation if the elderly differ from younger families with respect to income and the type of housing they demand.

The discussion raises issues which call for validation in future empirical research. A simulation model, as the one discussed in this paper, cannot provide information about the relative importance of the different processes responsible for changes in the demographic ecology. In particular, it cannot predict the results from the competition between the segregating influence of preferences and the market and the integrating influences of demographic processes and mobility. The empirical research surveyed in the second section did not provide an answer to this question. The various studies discussed concentrate on the joint effect of both sets of factors and ignore the countervailing contribution of the different processes. An understanding of these influences requires an in-depth analysis of empirical data, preferably within the context of a full econometric model of the housing market.

NOTES

1. This assumption is less restrictive than it appears. Suppose that the housing market is in equilibrium and all households are homogeneous regarding income and preferences. Differences between the willingness to pay for dissimilar dwelling units would then be exactly offset by rents, and households would be indifferent between units which differ with regard to quality and location.

2. The model could, without affecting the conclusions, be extended to include ability to pay, housing quality and endogenous rents (Werczberger, 1992). However, our purpose is to clarify the effect of mobility and structural aging on the demographic ecology. Therefore the complexity of a full economic housing market model did not seem to be justified by the additional realism gained.

3. Equation (13) is thus simplified to

$$X^t_{iab} = S^t_{iab} + \Sigma_j(M^t_{ja} + F^t_{ja})\, V^t_{ib}/\Sigma_{ib}V^t_{ib}, \qquad \text{all i, all b}$$

4. In a monocentric urban area, zones can be ordered by their distance d_i to the CBD, so that $i'' > i'$ implies $d_{i'} < d_{i''}$. Let P^t_i be the number of units required to meet the demand for housing in zone i and beyond (i.e., all zones $j \mid d_j > d_i$), after all vacant land in $k \mid d_k < d_i$ has been developed. Then

$$P^t_i = \Sigma_{ja}D^t_{ja} - \Sigma_{ib}[W^t_{ib} + U^t_{ib}] - \Sigma_{j\,<\,i}H^t_j \qquad \text{all i}$$

P^t_i thus equals the difference between $\Sigma_a D^t_a$, the total demand for vacant housing, $\Sigma_{ib}[W^t_{ib} + U^t_{ib}]$, the supply of surviving vacant dwellings and $\Sigma_{j\,<\,i}H^t_i$, the new units built in zones for which $d_j < d_i$. Vacant land suitable for construction in every zone is denoted by L^t_i. It equals the difference between q_i, the total capacity of the zone i, and the land taken by occupied dwelling units, i.e., which are not being demolished.

$$L^t_i = q_i - h_i\Sigma_{a'b'c_{b'}}X^{t'}_{ia'b'} \qquad \text{all i}$$

The coefficient h_i equals here the inverse density, which may vary by zone. Construction H^t_i is then computed iteratively for every zone i, starting with $i = 1$, the zone next to the CBD, and continuing to the most distant zone I.

$$\text{If } L^t_i/h_i < P^t_i \longrightarrow H^t_i = L^t_i/h_i \qquad \text{all t, all i}$$

$$\text{If } L^t_i/h_i \geq P^t_i \longrightarrow H^t_i = P^t_i \qquad \text{all t, all i}$$

If P^t_i, the new construction needed in zone i and beyond, exceeds what can be built in i, all vacant land in i will be used. Otherwise, construction in i just equals P^t_i.

5. Reluctance to move into more distant neighborhoods has the same effect as a lower propensity to move, as it tends to slow down spatial integration and to maintain spatial segregation.

6. Specifically, the algorithm proceeds as follows

(1) Let Q^{ts}_{ijab} be the probability that a moving household of type (j,a) prefers a vacant dwelling of type (i,b) in iteration s. It is calculated by substituting the current number of vacant dwellings VV^{ts}_{ib} (instead of V^t_{ib}) into equation (12).

(2) Estimate excess demand E^{ts}_{ib} for dwellings of type (i,b) as the difference between the supply VV^{ts}_{ib} and the total potential demand from each type of moving households for (i,b).

$$\Sigma_{ja}(Q^{ts}_{ijab}DD^{ts}_{ja}) - VV^{ts}_{ib} = E^{ts}_{ib} \qquad \text{all s, all i, all b (B.1)}$$

If there is no excess demand, i.e., if $E^{ts}_{ib} \leq 0$, all households which prefer to live in (ib) are assigned to one of the vacant dwellings. The remaining vacant dwellings are obtained from

$$VV^{ts+1}_{ib} = VV^{ts}_{ib} - \Sigma_{aj}(Q^{ts}_{ijab}DD^{ts}_{ja}) \qquad \text{all s, all i, all b (B.2)}$$

(3b) However, if there is excess demand, i.e., if $E^{ts}_{ib} > 0$, moving households are assigned to vacant dwellings in proportion to the ratio between the supply of vacant dwellings of type (i,b) and the total potential demand for (i,b).

$$X^{ts+1}_{iab} = X^t_{iab} + \Sigma_{ja}DD^{ts}_{ja}*Q^{ts}_{ijab}*[VV^{ts}_{ib}/\Sigma_{ja}(Q^{ts}_{ijab}DD^{ts}_{ja})]$$

$$\text{all s, all i, all b (B.3)}$$

No vacancies of type (i,b) are then left. The number of remaining moving households is

$$DD^{ts+1}_{ja} = DD^{ts}_{ja} - \Sigma_{ja}DD^{ts}_{ja}*Q^{ts}_{ijab}*[VV^{ts}_{ib}/\Sigma_{ja}(Q^{ts}_{ijab}DD^{ts}_{ja})]$$

$$\text{all s, all i, all b (B.4)}$$

(4) Convergence has been reached when all households have been assigned to a vacant dwelling, so that

$$\Sigma_{ja}DD^{ts+1}_{ja} = 0 \qquad \text{all s, all j (B.5)}$$

If $\Sigma_{ja}DD^{ts+1}_{ja} > 0$, the algorithm proceeds to the next iteration s + 1 and returns to step 1.

BIBLIOGRAPHY

Baer, W.C. and C.B. Williamson (1986). "The Filtering of Households and Housing Units." *Journal of Planning Literature* 3:2, 127-152.

Brueckner, Jan (1977). "The Determinants of Residential Succession." *Journal of Urban Economics*, 45-59.

Champion, A.G. (1989). "United Kingdom: Population Deconcentration as a Cyclic Phenomenon." In A.G. Champion (ed.), *Counterurbanization: The Changing Pace and Nature of Population Deconcentration*. London: Arnold.

Downs, A. (1981). *Neighborhood and Urban Development*. Washington: Brookings.

Golant, S. (1975). "Residential Concentration of the Future Elderly." *Gerontologist* 15:1, 16-23.

Grigsby, W.G. et al. (1987). *The Dynamics of Neighborhood Change and Decline*. Oxford: Pergamon.

Huttman, E. and E. Gurewitsch (1987). "The Elderly and Housing." In E. Huttman and W. van Vliet (eds.), *Handbook of Housing and the Built Environment in the United States*. N.Y.: Greenwood Press.

Lawton, M.P. and M.H. Kleban (1973). "The Inner-City Resident: To Move or Not to Move." *Gerontologist* 13, 443-448.

Lowry, I.S. (1960). "Filtering and Housing Standards: A Conceptual Analysis." *Land Economics* 36:4, 362-370.

Lowry, I.S. (1964). *A Model of Metropolis*. Santa Monica, CA: The Rand Corporation, RM-4125-RC.

Mattsson, L.G. (1984). "Equivalence Between Welfare and Entropy Approaches to Residential Location." *Regional Science and Urban Economics* 14, 147-173.

Newcomer, P. et al. (ed.) (1986). *Housing an Aging Society*. N.Y.: Van Nostrand.

Pampel, F.C. and H.M. Choldin (1978). "Urban Location and Segregation of the Aged: A Block Level Analysis." *Social Forces* 56:4, 1121-1139.

Rogers, A. (1989). "Elderly Mobility Transition: Growth, Concentration and Tenure." *Research on Aging* 11:1, 3-32.

Smith, B.W. and J. Hiltner (1975). "Intraurban Location of the Elderly." *Journal of Gerontology* 30:4, 473-478.

Spear, A. and J.W. Meyer (1988). "Types of Elderly Residential Mobility and Their Determinants." *Journal of Gerontology* 43:3, 574-581.

Werczberger, E. (1992). "Demographic Aging and the Spatial Structure of Urban Areas." Paper presented at the 32nd European Conference of the RSA in Louvain, Belgium, August 1992.

Wiseman, R.F. (1986). "Reconcentration and Migration of Older Americans." In Newcomer (ed.), *Housing an Aging Society*. N.Y.: Van Nostrand.

APPENDIX A

THE MATHEMATICAL FORMULATION OF THE MODEL

A.1 Notation

Consider an urban area divided into I zones, denoted by $i = 1, \ldots I$. Time is represented by discrete periods identified by t, $t = 1, \ldots T$. Changes in stock, such as construction and relocation occur at the beginning of each period. State variables represent conditions after these transitions have taken place.

The population consists of households which are homogeneous, except for age. There are A age groups denoted by $a = 1, \ldots A$. In every period, households are created, change residence and dissolve at exogenous, age-specific rates. Three coefficients define the respective probabilities. (1) The "rate of reproduction" of new households, g_a, is defined as the probability that a new household is created in period t for any household of age a existing in period $t - 1$. New households are taken to be young, so that their age is $a = 1$. (2) The survival rate d_a is the proportion of households of age a, which survive after the beginning of a period. The term $(1 - d_a)$ therefore equals the probability that households of age a dissolve. (3) The mobility rate m_a is the proportion of households of age a, which change residence at the beginning of each period. Its value is taken to be independent of the household's previous moving experience.

All dwelling units are assumed to be of equal size and built with the same initial characteristics. They age without changing quality and are demolished when maintenance costs become excessive. There are B building age groups, denoted by $b = 1, \ldots B$. The coefficient c_b equals the proportion of surviving units of age b, i.e., of units which are not demolished at the beginning of a period.

A solution of the model consists of a vector $\{X^t_{iab}\}$, whose generic element X^t_{iab} equals the number of households of age a, which live in period t and zone i in a dwelling of age b. To simplify the notation, an apostrophe is used to denote the indices $t - 1$, $a - 1$ and $b - 1$, by t', a' and b', respectively.

A.2 The Demand for Vacant Dwellings

Demand for vacant dwellings originates from three sources: new households, households which relocate voluntarily, and those forced to move because of the demolition of their dwelling.

New households: The number of new households N^t in period t is obtained as the weighted sum of the different age groups in the preceding period t', where the weights equal the age-specific "reproduction rate" $g_{a'}$.

$$N^t = \Sigma_{ia'b'}g_{a'}X^{t'}_{ia'b'} \tag{1}$$

Voluntary relocation: M^t_{ja} is the number of surviving households of age a in zone j, which relocate for personal reasons such as a change in size or income.

$$M^t_{ja} = \Sigma_b(d_{a'}c_{b'}m_a)X^{t'}_{ja'b'} \qquad \text{all j, all a} \tag{2}$$

The expression $(d_{a'}c_{b'}m_{a'})$ in (2) is the product of three terms, which equal, respectively, the survival rate of households of age a' and of the dwelling of age b' and the probability of voluntary relocation.

Demolition: Equation (3) defines F^t_{ja}, the number of households living in j, that relocate because of the demolition of their dwelling.

$$F^t_{ja} = \Sigma_{b'}d_{a'}(1 - c_{b'})X^{t'}_{ja'b'} \qquad \text{all j, all a} \tag{3}$$

Total demand: The demand D^t_{ja} for vacant dwellings by households relocating from j is defined differently according to the age of the households.

$$D^t_{*1} = N^t \qquad \text{for a} = 1 \tag{4a}$$

$$D^t_{ja} = M^t_{ja} + F^t_{ja} \qquad \text{for a} > 1 \tag{4b}$$

Since new households have no zone of origin, we substitute in (4a) an asterisk (*) for $a = 1$ instead of the subscript j in D^t_{ja}. For older households total demand is simply the sum of the two mover categories.

The number of surviving households S^t_{iab}, which continue to live in the same dwelling as in the previous period, is then given by

$$S^t_{iab} = d_{a'}c_{b'}(1 - m_{a'})X^{t'}_{ia'b'} \qquad \text{all i, all a, all b} \tag{5}$$

A.3 The Supply of Vacant Dwellings

Vacant housing is provided from three sources: dissolution of existing households, relocation, and new construction.

Household dissolution: W^t_{ib}, the number of dwellings of age b in i that are vacant because of the dissolution of households, is obtained from

$$W^t_{ib} = \Sigma_{a'}[(1 - d_{a'})c_{b'}]X^{t'}_{ia'b'} \qquad \text{all i, all b} \qquad (6)$$

Relocation: Dwelling units, which are vacant because of relocation, are denoted by U^t_{ib}. They are obtained from expression (2) by summing over household age instead of over building age.

$$U^t_{ib} = \Sigma_{a'}[d_{a'}c_{b'}m_{a'}]X^{t'}_{ia'b'} \qquad \text{all i, all b} \qquad (7)$$

New construction: Total construction in any period t, $\Sigma_i H^t_i$, equals the demand for new housing, given demolition and net growth in the number of households. If dwellings remain vacant in any period, they are demolished. To obtain the location of new construction, all employment and services are assumed to be concentrated in the center. More centrally located areas are therefore preferred to more peripheral ones and will be developed first. The algorithm used scans all zones in order of their distance from the center, and allocates new construction to more distant locations, only when no vacant land is left closer to the CBD.[4]

The total number of vacant dwellings of age b in zone i is V^t_{ib}. It is the sum of three terms: W^t_{ib}, vacancies due to the dissolution of a household; U^t_{ib}, vacancies created by relocation; and H^t_i, the newly constructed and thus vacant units.

$$V^t_{ib} = W^t_{ib} + U^t_{ib} + H^t_i \qquad \text{all i, all b} \qquad (8)$$

A.4 Location Preferences

Location preferences of moving households are simulated using an age-specific linear stochastic utility function (9). The utility of the choice of a dwelling unit is then the function of variables, which account for the behavioral characteristics of the elderly, such as distance of move and spatial externalities. In the present version, only proximity to other elderly or services is included as argument of the utility function.[5]

Expression (9) defines the total utility $U^{*t}_a(i,j,b)$, of a household of age a living in zone j, which decides to move in period t and selects alternative (i,b).

$$U^{*t}_a(i,j,b) = f_a(Y^{t'}_{i'a'}) + \varepsilon_{ijab} \qquad \text{all i, all j, all a, all b} \qquad (9)$$

The first element of (9), $f_a(Y^{t'}_{i'a'})$, equals the utility associated with living in a zone, in which the proportion or density of households of age a' equals $Y^t_{i'a'}$, where $Y^t_{i'a'} = (\Sigma_{b'}X^{t'}_{ia'b'}/\Sigma_{a'b'}X^{t'}_{ia'b'})$. In general, we would assume that $f_a(.)$ is an increasing function of $Y^t_{i'a'}$, the proportion of households of age a, but that its value is negligible, except for the elderly. The last term in (10) is the Weibull distributed stochastic error ε_{iab}. It may be generated by unobserved location factors, variations in building quality or taste differences among households.

The expected or systematic utility of a choice (i,b) involving i and b is obtained by omitting the error term ε_{iab}.

$$U^t_{ijab} = f_a(Y^{t'}_{i'a'}) \qquad \text{all i, all a, all b} \quad (10)$$

A household will choose alternative (i,b) if the implied total utility is greater than or equal to the utility of any alternative $(i',b')|i' \neq i, b' \neq b)$. Let Q^t_{ijab} denote the probability that a household of age a which resides in period t in j chooses alternative (i,b). Q^t_{ijab} is then proportional to U^t_{ijab}, the utility associated with the choice, as well as to V^t_{ib}, the supply of vacant dwellings of age b in zone i (McFadden, 1973; Snickars and Wei-bull, 1977). The probability of choosing (i,b) is

$$Q^t_{ijab} = V^t_{ib}\exp(\mu U^t_{ijab})/\Sigma_{ib}V^t_{ib}\exp(\mu U^t_{ijab}) \quad \text{all i, all a, all b} \quad (11)$$

The parameter μ is a constant and equal for all i, a and b, so that it can be omitted (Mattsson, 1984). Substituting (10) into (11) yields a probabilistic choice model for the representative household.

$$Q^t_{ijab} = \frac{V^t_{ib}\exp[f_a(Y^t_{i'a'})]}{\Sigma_{i''a''b''}V^t_{i''b''}\exp[f_a(Y^t_{i'a'})]} \qquad (12)$$

A.5 Allocation of Moving Households to Dwellings

Households are assigned to vacant dwellings using a modification of the Lowry model (Lowry, 1964). At the beginning of every iteration, denoted by the superscripts $= 1, 2,..$, two vectors are computed: the vector DD^{ts}_{ja} of moving households, not yet allocated to a dwelling, and the vector of vacant dwellings VV^{ts}_{ib}. Hence, in the first iteration, s = 1 and $DD^{t1}_{ja} = D^t_{ja}$, for all j and a, and $VV^{t1}_{ib} = V^t_{ib}$, for all i and b.

Using equation (12), moving households are then temporarily assigned to their preferred choice (i,b) among the vacant dwellings. If there is no excess demand for alternative (i,b), all households are assigned to (i,b) and added to the current vector X^{ts}_{iab}. If there is excess demand for (i,b), the proportion of households assigned to (i,b) equals the ratio of the supply of vacant dwellings of that type and the total demand for it.

In the next iteration s + 1, the same method is used to assign the remaining households, which have not yet been allocated. This process is continued until all movers have been assigned to a vacant dwelling.

The total number of households X^t_{iab} of age a in units of age b in any zone i in period t is then the sum of, S^t_{iab}, the surviving households, who remained in their dwelling, and of those who moved or were assigned to a vacant dwelling at the beginning of period t by the allocation procedure described above.[6]

Chapter 10

Regulation and Evaluation Criteria for Housing for the Elderly: An International Comparison

Ernest R. Alexander

SUMMARY. Housing for the elderly is subject to regulation in most countries. The types of housing that should be subject to regulation are discussed, including issues to be addressed by regulation, such as the interdependence between location and services, and the implications of continuous occupancy. Regulatory regimes in Germany, Israel, the Netherlands, the U.K. and the U.S.A. are described and compared, to suggest the dimensions of the ideal regulatory framework. Criteria for evaluating elderly housing proposals are developed, and this paper presents an evaluation system for use in the regulatory review of congregate housing and small nursing home projects. *[Article copies available for a fee from The Haworth Document Delivery Service: 1-800-342-9678. E-mail address: getinfo@haworth.com]*

INTRODUCTION

Like all housing, housing for the elderly is subject to regulation in most countries. The statutory framework of regulation varies from country to

Ernest R. Alexander, PhD, is affiliated with The Public Policy Program, Tel-Aviv University, Tel-Aviv 69978, Israel.

[Haworth co-indexing entry note]: "Regulation and Evaluation Criteria for Housing for the Elderly: An International Comparison." Alexander, Ernest R. Co-published simultaneously in *Journal of Housing for the Elderly* (The Haworth Press, Inc.) Vol. 12, No. 1/2, 1997, pp. 147-168; and: *Shelter and Service Issues for Aging Populations: International Perspectives* (ed: Leon A. Pastalan) The Haworth Press, Inc., 1997, pp. 147-168. Single or multiple copies of this article are available for a fee from The Haworth Document Delivery Service [1-800-342-9678, 9:00 a.m. - 5:00 p.m. (EST). E-mail address: getinfo@haworth.com].

country, as do the institutions that develop the regulations and apply them. One of the ways in which regulation of housing for the elderly can differ is whether there are any special regulations or procedures that apply to housing for the elderly in particular, as distinct from any other types of housing or construction.

In Israel, the building regulations that apply to housing for the elderly are identical to those applying to any other residential construction.[1] This situation stimulated the study presented here, when it became apparent that the lack of regulatory criteria distinguishing between housing for the elderly and ordinary residential construction was subject to abuse.[2] The aim of the study was to define the types of housing which should be subject to special consideration, and develop criteria for evaluating plans that were submitted as housing for the elderly.[3] The study includes a review of regulation of housing for the elderly in Israel, Germany, the Netherlands, the U.K. and the U.S.A., and concludes with an evaluation framework that was recommended for reviewing plans for housing for the elderly in the context of Israel's statutory system of land development control.

For the purposes of the study, it was necessary to identify and define housing for the elderly and distinguish it from other residential construction. This is not a trivial issue, since the elderly are in fact housed in ways that vary along a wide continuum. At one pole of this range is ordinary housing that differs from any other housing only in its age-specific occupants; at the other extreme are geriatric wards that provide housing to their elderly patients incidentally to their medical care. Even housing that is not planned specially for use by elderly residents may serve distinct age-differentiated populations, as happens in the "naturally occurring retirement communities" found where there are high concentrations of elderly populations, as for example in Florida.

To determine the types of housing that would be included in this study's terms of reference, the housing stock was divided into two main groups: ordinary housing in the community, and housing planned for use by the elderly. When the latter is designed for elderly residents whose entitlement is based on their age, but they are still functionally independent (e.g., some subsidized Section 8 housing in the U.S., and some public housing in Israel), then for regulatory purposes such housing can be included with the former group, i.e., it would be regulated just like all other housing.

The dwelling types specially planned and designed for use by the elderly vary with their residents' degree of independence, or their functional impairment or disability. They range from non-institutional through semi-institutional to completely institutional housing. Under non-institutional housing we find *retirement communities*, which may occupy part of a neighborhood, a whole neighborhood, or even be complete self-contained settlements. These are designed primarily for independent elderly, are made up mainly of single-family units, but they may also include other types of housing for the elderly described below. Retirement communities vary widely in their size, from around 100 units at the lowest extreme to over 10,000 units. They also vary in their array of facilities and the packages of services they offer, which include various combinations of health facilities and medical services, recreation facilities and other services (Marans, Hunt and Vakalo, 1984).

Semi-institutional housing includes *sheltered or congregate housing*, which has been defined as a non-institutional residential setting adapted to the special needs of the elderly by appropriate design and the provision of selected supportive services (Monk and Kaye, 1991). Sheltered or congregate housing may be made up of dwelling units which are dispersed in a neighborhood, but they are more usually clustered around their common facilities or the source of services. The kinds of layout of sheltered housing for the elderly vary widely, but all have a central core which includes areas for common social activities, special functions and services, or the dwelling units are linked to a separate facility which contains the same spaces and provides the services. The residents of congregate or sheltered housing are relatively independent elderly who have minimal functional impairment (Chellis, Seagle and Seagle, 1982).

Institutional housing includes nursing homes, geriatric centers, and geriatric wards in hospitals. *Nursing homes* ("boarding homes" in the U.K.) provide group housing and domiciliary care in rooms, or suites with limited housekeeping facilities, for less independent elderly who need more intensive supportive services. The services nursing homes provide can range from domiciliary care and housekeeping through limited health care up to relatively continuous nursing care and medical services, but by definition, nursing homes occupy the less institutionalized end of the spectrum. They try to convey a domestic rather than an institutional ambience (though some are quite large) and the majority of their residents are somewhat independent and not so functionally impaired as to require continuous nursing care. In size, nursing homes can range from as few as ten to hundreds of units.

The *geriatric center* is usually a large multifunctional complex that combines several or all of the housing types reviewed here. In particular, the geriatric center is distinguished from the nursing home by its much larger proportion of residents who need continuous nursing care and intensive supportive services. Geriatric centers may be affiliated with and linked to hospitals and then they will include geriatric and psycho-geriatric wards.

This range of types of housing for the elderly opens up the question of the relevant subject of regulation. Since the point of departure was the distinction between ordinary residential construction and housing for the elderly, we need not be concerned with patently institutional housing: large nursing homes, geriatric centers, and geriatric wards in hospitals. All these, with their significant component of health care and medical services, fall under a somewhat different regulatory regime. Consequently, the focus here is on housing for the elderly in the form of sheltered or congregate housing and smaller nursing homes.

There are two other issues concerning housing for the elderly, which may affect regulatory intervention: the relation between location and services, and the fit between dwelling units and their elderly residents over time.

Location and services: one of the aspects characterising housing for the elderly is its residents' dependence on specific services. These vary in their importance for different housing types, according to the relative independence or functional impairment of their aging residents. In order of their respective priority, we can identify the following services:

Monitoring and communication; security and alarm; housekeeping and maintenance of the dwelling units and of common facilities and areas; social, cultural and recreational activities; food service and provision of meals; personal services (laundry, home-help, etc.); health services (pharmacy, clinic, etc.); community services (day center, religious facilities, welfare and social services); shopping and commercial services (bank, drugstore and beautician/cosmetics, travel agency, etc.); urban services and amenities (post office, park, shopping center, cafe/restaurant, cultural facilities: library, theatre, concert hall, etc.).

According to their relative independence or impairment, various groups of elderly residents need different packages of these services and have changing priorities. Thus, as their functional capacity and mobility declines, they will be less interested in access to community services and urban amenities. At the same time, their personal service needs will be more urgent, they will become more dependent on supportive services, and the availability of health care and medical services will become critical (Altman, Lawton and Wohlwill, 1984).

There is also a trade-off between site-based service provision and access to services at other locations. Accordingly, a minimum set of services has to be defined that must be delivered on-site for each type of housing for the elderly. The remaining services, according to their relative priority, can either be provided on-site or be available elsewhere as needed. The implication of these service needs, for regulation of housing for the elderly, is that location of the housing in the urban context is critical, though to the degree that there is a wider array of in-house services, location and accessibility of outside services becomes less important.

Continuous occupancy and its implications: as noted above, the elderly differ significantly in their relative independence and functional impairment. As they age, they can pass through the stages of relative independence, through increasing frailty, to high degrees of functional and psychological impairment and dependence. Each of these stages poses changing demands on the occupant's residential setting and wider urban environment, and has different service needs. The aging process, then, raises the problem of the fit between the elderly occupants' needs and their housing. There are several ways of addressing this problem.

The "adaptive" approach offers housing types, each of which is maximally adapted to its intended occupants' specific needs. Their residential settings, then, remain constant, but as their functional and mental condition changes, the aging residents move to other, more appropriate housing. This approach has the merits of efficiency and providing the optimal setting for each elderly resident, at relatively low cost. Its drawback is the separation of residents from their homes, sometimes more than once, during the latter part of their lifetimes. This can be a traumatic experience, which it is better to avoid.

The "responsive" approach recognizes this problem, and provides one continuous dwelling unit. The design of this unit maximises flexibility, so as to make the housing as responsive as possible to its elderly residents' needs at different stages of their aging process. Flexibility of the housing complex's service infrastructure is also essential, so that a rich and changing array of services is available to meet residents' changing demands. While ensuring permanent housing, this approach also has its flaws. The difficulty of offering an optimal setting for each stage of the resident's occupancy in the same dwelling, and the high costs of flexibility raise the temptation to effect savings by limiting adaptiveness.

A third way tries to combine both these approaches, by providing a variety of housing types in a common setting (one building or a complex of buildings on one site) under continuous single management. This has the advantages of the "adaptive" approach, but reduces the trauma of residents' moving by retaining the comfort of familiar surroundings. This has become a widespread response among housing providers to the elderly, who want to commit their residents to long-term contracts. Continuous residence and services through the duration of the aging process are provided in geriatric centers that combine congregate housing, domiciliary care and nursing home wings, and geriatric wards in one complex under unified management (Hunt, 1991).

In the context of planning regulation of housing for the elderly, this issue raises the question: How can housing be encouraged that provides continuity of occupancy, and offers the changing array of services its aging residents will need?[4] In the absence of any such commitment to elderly occupants by the housing provider, there is the risk that as they grow older, some residents may need facilities and services that are not covered under their original contracts, and end up as a burden on local governments' social services.

REGULATING HOUSING FOR THE ELDERLY

In Israel, planning regulation of housing for the elderly is under the same hierarchical system of statutory planning and development control as all landuses and types of construction (Alexander, Alterman and Law-Yone, 1983). The Israeli planning system is administered by Town Planning and Building Commissions at the local and District levels, and exceptional projects are also subject to review and approval by the National Planning and Building Council and sign off by the Minister of the Interior.

Two other agencies participate in regulation of housing for the elderly. Through its statutory jurisdiction over operation of "hostels" for "dependent individuals," the Ministry of Labor and Welfare licences the operation of any housing for the elderly that has more than ten units.[5] Besides prescribing operating procedures, the applicable regulations include minimum standards applying to some aspects of planning and building design. For example, they require elevators (and prescribe their minimum size) for multistorey housing, and they indicate that pavillion-type housing must be linked by enclosed passages of no less than 1.80m width (Ministry of Labor and Welfare, 1986).

Any facility providing health care or medical services must also have a permit from the Ministry of Health. This applies to hospitals, and also covers congregate housing for the elderly and nursing homes that provide any health care services. The Ministry of Health's detailed manual of operating regulations also specifies space requirements and standards for equipment and finishes for areas housing identified health-related functions, such as physicians' examination rooms, physiotherapy rooms, nursing stations, etc. (Ministry of Health, 1991).

State subsidised housing for the elderly is subject to oversight by the Ministry of Construction and Housing, which has issued standards (Ministry of Construction and Housing, 1991) that are mandatory on such housing and also frequently used by other sponsors as design guidelines. Planning guidelines for nursing homes have also been published by the Israel Lands Administration (1991).[6]

On the face of it, then, housing for the elderly in Israel is not underregulated. On the contrary, perhaps the complaints of some developers of housing projects for the elderly, that they are overregulated, are warranted. But closer examination exposes some significant gaps in the regulatory system. There is no planning control of housing for the elderly as such, and there is little or no coordination between the planning process, and the functional licencing and permitting systems.[7] These gaps have several consequences. One is neglect of the locational aspects of housing for the elderly. Another is exploitation of the disjunction between the planning and permitting processes by unscrupulous developers. These ask for (and have received) planning permission for subsequent changes in landuse (e.g., from approved housing for the elderly to conventional multifamily housing or to an apartment hotel) on the claim that they were unable to get their expected operating permits from the other regulatory agencies. The procedures and evaluation criteria recommended below are designed to address and correct these deficiencies.

At the opposite extreme of Israel's centralized hierarchical systems of control is the U.S.A., where planning and land use regulation is delegated (by the States) to the local level, where it is implemented at widely varying degrees of consistency and permissiveness (Cullingworth, 1993). The local zoning plans and ordinances which are the main land development control tool usually make no distinction between housing for the elderly and any other type of residential land use. However, it appears that projects proposing housing for the elderly may often meet the criteria for planned unit development[8] so that they become the subjects of a more flexible approval process.

Though there has been a proliferation of design guides for housing for the elderly (Valins, 1982; Carstens, 1985; Regnier and Pynoos, 1987), no formal or uniform standards have been developed at the federal level. The only exception to this applies to housing projects that enjoy federal subsidy, which have to conform to Federal Housing Administration (1966) issued minimum standards. In the relevant functional areas of welfare and health services and medical facilities, which also apply to some housing for the elderly such as nursing homes, State agencies exercise control by licencing and monitoring, but the interstate variation in regulatory effectiveness is notorious.[9]

The cumulative result of all these factors is that the U.S. (in varying degrees among its States) offers the project developer or sponsor of housing for the elderly a regulatory environment that is probably unparalleled for its permissiveness and range for individual discretion. Leaving planning, design and development decisions to be primarily determined by market considerations, which is the prevailing regulatory philosophy in the U.S., has advantages in promoting diversity, creativity, and responsiveness to manifest demand, but also risks abuse.

Germany, as a federal republic, does not differ much from the U.S.A. in its planning control of housing for the elderly, although formal land development regulation in Germany is considerably more developed than in the U.S., and employs a substantial bureaucracy. The German *Land* fills the same role as the American State; consequently, in Germany there is the same absence of central control that there is in the U.S., and planning control and sectoral regulation are decentralized to the Länder. However, unlike the U.S., some Federal ministries undertake active sponsorship of research and evaluation of housing for the elderly and issue design and operating guidelines.[10]

Britain is more like Israel in its centralized system of planning and development control, but regulation of housing for the elderly has gone through several significant changes. Like other facilities delivering health services, nursing homes which provide supportive services and health care are regulated by the Ministry of Health and its agencies. Sheltered housing for the elderly, like all housing and other building, is regulated by the Department of the Environment (previously, the Ministry of Housing and Local Government), but in effect, planning permission for all but exceptional projects is subject to local authorities' control.

Housing for the elderly which was publicly subsidised (which included "Council Housing" built by local authorities) had to conform to standards for sheltered housing for the elderly (Ministry of Housing and Local Government, 1969), which were also used as guidelines by local authorities for their planning review of privately sponsored projects. But in the Thatcher government's deregulation campaign, these standards were withdrawn in 1982, and since then local authorities have been free to review and approve proposed housing for the elderly at their discretion. Currently, the only criterion the Department of the Environment requires local authorities to apply to projects involving public funding is whether their benefits warrant the expenditure.[11] Standards for housing the elderly are also included in an advisory circular issued by the Department of the Environment and Department of Health (1992).

The Netherlands is another country with a well developed hierarchical system of land use and development planning and control (Faludi and v.d.

Valk, 1994). This system extends from the national level (with strategic sectoral plans and a national physical development policy) through the Provinces, whose statutory plans (*streekplanne*) control local development to a significant degree, to the local level where each jurisdiction has its binding land use and development plan (*bestemmingsplan*). Nursing homes are regulated by the Ministry of Social Services and Welfare and the Ministry of Health, and national welfare policy also devotes attention to housing for the elderly in general.

The Ministry of Housing, Spatial Order and the Environment, or VROM (*Ministerium van Volkshuisvesting, Ruimtelijke Ordening en Milieu*) implements national policy regarding new housing construction through funding allocations to the various classes of subsidised housing (which include housing for the elderly). In this capacity, VROM sets standards for planning, design and construction for all housing built with public support, which are published annually in regulations (*Niewbouwregeling*), and construction codes (*Bouwbesluit*) that are issued periodically. Local governments are also required to develop their own plans for housing for the elderly (*ouderenhuis-vestingsplan*) according to VROM issued guidelines.

It is clear from the above that housing for the elderly in the Netherlands is highly regulated, and that public policy has a major impact on housing for the elderly and its related services. For example, recent regulations have addressed the problem of continuity of occupancy discussed above, by encouraging housing in larger multifunctional geriatric centers (VROM, 1991).

This brief review of how housing for the elderly is regulated in some countries does not offer any startling revelations. No one regulatory structure or procedure is clearly superior, and the wide variation between countries is less attributable to deliberate design than to history. Though perhaps the downsides of more permissive approaches, in the form of abuses that exploit gaps in regulations or interagency coordination, are more apparent, the shortcomings of more regulation cannot be ignored: oppressive bureaucracy that raises housing costs by imposing unnecessary requirements and delays, and restrictive rules that stifle diversity and limit consumer choice.

The ideal system of public control of housing for the elderly would consist of a minimal framework of regulation. Some regulation is necessary to avoid exploitation of market failures, such as consumer ignorance, as in the problem of ensuring continuity of occupancy and care for elderly residents. Planning control is necessary to effect the coordination of producers' decisions that the "free" market cannot, for example, preventing nuisances and undesirable external effects on elderly housing by incompatible adjacent land uses, or avoiding locations where elderly residents lack access to services they need. At the same time, such a system should cut the regulatory burden and facilitate the permitting process, by enabling sponsors and developers of housing for the elderly to obtain approval for their plans in a one-stop procedure that involves all the supervising agencies.

EVALUATION CRITERIA

The criteria for evaluating plans for housing for the elderly, which are presented below, are intended to reflect positive attributes of the relevant housing types, or respond to requirements such housing must meet if it is to be responsive to its residents' needs. There is a body of research that offers some empirical evidence of what these requirements are, and some of them are already incorporated in standards that have been developed for guidance or regulatory purposes.

Since these criteria are designed for use in plan assessment and review, they only address those aspects of the projected housing for the elderly that are under the purview of the planning and development control authority. These are also the aspects on which the submitted plans provide information or the evaluating official can obtain the needed data, either from available sources or by requiring supplementary information from the applicant.

These aspects include:

Location: where the proposed sheltered housing development or nursing home is located. This is important from several points of view. At the micro- to meso-scale, location is related to the potential for nuisances or negative externalities between incompatible adjoining or nearby landuses; this is reflected in some of the criteria developed below. At the macro-scale, location relates to the spatial distribution of relevant facilities and services in the project's urban setting, which (together with infrastructure characteristics, such as the street pattern, and transportation services, such as public transit) determines the elderly residents' access to needed services and desired urban amenities.

Site: several site characteristics address criteria which reflect a project's performance. Information on the size, shape, and topography of the site enables assessment of land coverage and setback criteria, of whether the planned layout offers site development and landscaping that provide appropriate open space and recreational amenities, and enables adequate vehicular circulation and pedestrian access compatible with mobility limitations of its elderly population. Site characteristics include microclimate (sun, wind and weather directions as affected by orientation and topography), which has a bearing on the quality of recreational open space and semi-enclosed spaces created by the building layout.

Layout: the form, juxtaposition, and massing of the proposed structure or buildings combine with the site information to enable application of planning regulations and several other criteria presented below. Some of these address the proposal's compatibility with its adjoining urban fabric and built environment. This is an important dimension in evaluating types of housing for the elderly that aim to minimize their institutional associations and to enhance their residential character by blending with their neighborhood surroundings.

Building/s: planning review does not cover detailed building characteristics and construction (e.g., internal floor plans and construction details), but some information on building spaces and functions is necessary. In particular, this relates to conformity with functional agencies' (the Ministry of Labor and Welfare, and the Ministry of Health) regulations, which a rational regulatory system should integrate with planning control (see below). This information may be provided in the form of schematic plans, or it may be presented as a program describing the relevant functions, spaces, and their dimensions.

Location

Housing for the elderly that tries to retain a noninstitutional character, such as sheltered or congregate housing and smaller residential-style nursing homes, must be well integrated into the fabric of their urban setting, and blend in with the built environment of its neighborhood. This has implications for such projects' location, which will be addressed below, but which are less important for more institutionalized developments: large nursing homes and geriatric centers. Housing for the elderly must also occupy a heathful location without significant air or noise pollution.

Accessibility of services and amenities is an important attribute of housing for the elderly. A location that is near the relevant facilities, or that offers easy access by public transit, provides such accessibility. Some substitution between proximity and transportation convenience must also be taken into account.

Desirable accessibility to services is ranked according to the priority of the service and the frequency of its use. According to one proposed British standard, sheltered housing should not be further than 200m from the nearest bus stop or transit station, and 600m from a postal branch, pharmacy, and store. Other facilities which should be in walking distance include a post office, grocery, medical and dental clinic, branch bank, public garden or park, church, pub, and day center (Lawton, 1986).

Several American studies have ranked services according to their intensity (number of users and frequency of use) related to their relative distance from respondents' housing. Food stores and physicians are the most intensively used services (over 80%), and are located between one and ten blocks away. Between 60% and 70% of responding elderly used shops, churches, and banks located between four to six blocks away, 40% visit beauticians-cosmetics/drugstores one to three blocks from their homes, and about 30% go to restaurants, parks, and clubs. The least intensively used were recreational facilities and library, by only 18-19% of the respondents (Carstens, 1985).

Another proposal suggests the following distances between sheltered housing and its services: food store–650m, pharmacy–500m, public transit stop–500m, other commercial services (supermarket and clothing stores, bank, beautician, hairdresser, etc.)–650m, medical services–800m, restaurant and post office–1km. The location should also offer access to central urban amenities: community center, cultural facilities, commercial center and a medical center (Israel Land Administration, 1988).

Site

Sites for sheltered housing or small nursing homes should fit their intended uses from the following aspects:

Landuse: even though the main designated landuse will be housing for the elderly, the site may include other appropriate landuses, when multi-functional utilization of the site is beneficial both to the project's residents and to the surrounding community. For example, in a densely built-up central city location, a sheltered housing complex could include uses that will offer services to the residents of the development as well as to neighborhood residents: shopping, commercial and personal services, medical clinic, day center or community center, etc. At the same time, the possibility of multiple landuse designation of housing sites for the elderly should not open the door to inappropriate or incompatible landuses on the site, which would be sources of nuisance to the project's residents.

Area: the site must be large enough to accommodate the proposed building layout and program, and leave enough space for landscape development that gives the residents appropriate open space and recreational opportunities.

Topography: the site's topography must allow development of a road network that conforms to applicable standards and that provides vehicular access as needed, including access for emergency vehicles to every point that has pedestrian access. The site should also enable the development of pedestrian paths and walkways that give access to all areas designated for use (i.e., excluding nature areas or landscape elements designed solely for visual effect) for all residents, including those with limited mobility or wheelchair-confined. This implies that no grade of any walkway should exceed 5%, though in exceptional circumstances ramp connections are acceptable if their slope is no greater than 1:12 (8.33%) and their length does not exceed 10m.

Access and privacy: the site must enable easy vehicular and pedestrian access from the adjoining street. It is also desirable for the site's form and its location in relation to the surrounding neighborhood to support a building layout that enables clear distinction between "open" areas which can be used jointly by elderly residents of the complex and other neighborhood or community residents, and "private" areas that are limited for project residents' access and use.

Layout

Sheltered or congregate housing and nursing homes can be designed in a wide variety of building layouts, depending on the site, type of dwelling unit, and the surrounding area. Densities and building forms can vary significantly, and there is no evidence to indicate optimum densities for development, or any preferred building form. Indeed, some research suggests that these are not significant factors affecting elderly residents' satisfaction (Krupat, 1985). However, as noted above, for housing that is designed to downplay its institutional association, it is important for its layout to fit as well as possible with the built form and character of the surrounding neighborhood. Some issues related to layout are:

Size: there are some recommendations and standards that set limits to the sizes of sheltered housing projects. One suggestion (though, dating back to the '70s, it is perhaps somewhat obsolete) sets the optimal size of congregate housing at thirty units, and proposes a fifty unit maximum (Department of the Environment, 1974). Another proposes to define sheltered or congregate housing as a complex including no fewer than 25 and no more than 120 units (Israel Land Administration, 1988). Other guidelines, intended for subsidised housing in Israel, suggest a minimal size of 25 to 30 units, and an upper limit of 120 units for sheltered housing for the elderly (Ministry of Construction and Housing, 1991).

Setting a minimum number of units for sheltered housing or nursing homes serves the purpose of ensuring an adequate level of service and management, but there is no evidence to support the 25-unit threshold of these proposals. Amendments to the present regulations currently in preparation in the Ministry of Labor and Welfare propose a 10-unit minimum (based on limiting permit requirements to "hostels" with more than 13 residents); this seems reasonable.

It also appears that with time the norms of scale for congregate housing and nursing homes have changed, and much larger complexes of congregate housing and nursing homes are now acceptable if their layouts and form meet other relevant criteria. There is already congregate housing that includes over 700 units in one complex. We can conclude that the range of optimal size for sheltered or congregate housing developments for the elderly has broadened, and might span from a minimum of about 13 units to around a 500-unit maximum.

Roads and parking: vehicular access to the main entrance and other appropriate points (such as emergency entrances and loading dock) has to be provided by an internal road network that meets prevailing engineering and traffic standards, and emergency vehicle access to all places that are pedestrian-accessible is also essential. The pedestrian connection between the main vehicular access and the building entrance must be short and easy.

Adequate parking must be provided for residents', staff, service, and visitors' cars. Parking multipliers (number of spaces per resident, or per dwelling unit, or per unit of floorspace area of a specified function) can vary widely, depending on the location and the intended population of the housing. In Israel, one standard proposes 0.25 spaces per dwelling unit (Ministry of Construction and Housing, 1991). Some guidelines vary the multipliers systematically, depending on location and expected car-ownership, for example, U.S. and Canadian guidelines present multipliers varying from one place per 6 units for central-urban locations with superior service access and public transit (in Canada) to one place per four units (Canada) and one per unit (U.S.A.) for sites in rural locations or small towns with poor access to services and no public transit. For urban sites located in high density areas, it is particularly important to assign short-term parking for service and emergency vehicles, and visitors; one recommended multiplier for such parking proposes 6 spaces for complexes of up to 100 units, 10 for complexes between 101 and 200 units, and 12 for development over 200 units in size (Carstens, 1986).

Outside areas and open space: the layout of the housing should blend with the surrounding built environment. Design guidelines recommend close links between buildings' interior spaces and the outside, creating exterior areas in the form of balconies, terraces, or patios that are extensions of inside spaces. Exterior areas formed by the building layout should include sheltered and shaded sitting areas or nooks, landscaped areas and walkways. Sometimes there are also regulations prescribing some aspects of building layout; for example, in Israel, housing for the elderly that is designed in pavillion form must be connected by enclosed walkways that are not less than 1.80m wide (Ministry of Labor and Welfare, 1985).

Building/s: The building program and design is only relevant to planning review to the extent that it is prescribed by other regulating agencies. Where this is the case (as it is in Israel), this should become an integral part of plan review. For example, minimum programs for sheltered housing and nursing homes in Israel are included in the current and proposed regulations prescribing their operations. Information on some external building characteristics, such as materials and finishes, roofs, etc., may be necessary to judge the degree to which the project meets the criterion, suggested above, of consistency with its surrounding built environment.

CRITERIA AND PERFORMANCE MEASURES

The following criteria and their related performance measures make up an evaluation instrument that was developed for use in planning review of proposals for elderly housing in Israel. There are two kinds of criteria: critical criteria and optional criteria. A proposal's conformity with the critical criteria is measured on a dichotomous scale; i.e., it either meets the criterion or it does not. The critical criteria generally reflect existing regulations, and the proposed scoring method implies that failure to meet all of them will result in denial of approval for the project.

The optional criteria reflect important and desirable performance characteristics, and proposed plans are evaluated on their attainment of each criterion, and scored accordingly (on a 5-point scale). The weights assigned to these criteria reflect a subjective judgement, which plan reviewers or evaluating agencies can modify according to their particular assessment of the criteria's relative priorities. The final score is the weighted aggregation of a proposal's scores on all the criteria, and evaluators can decide (or be instructed) on their relative severity or permissiveness by setting a higher or lower threshold for plan approval. The final score is arrived at as follows:

$$F = 0.2 * \sum_{i=1}^{n} S_{ki} \sum_{j=1}^{n} W_{cj} S_{cj}$$

F: final score

S: score

c: criterion (optional)

k: criterion (critical)

W: weight (priority)

Location

K.1: Within Urban Fabric
The project must be located within the continuous urban fabric of a city or town.
Performance measure: If the site is surrounded on all sides or two or more sides by a built-up residential neighborhood–S = 1; if only one side of the site abuts a built-up residential neighborhood, or it is only linked to the urbanized area by one street, or it is on the edge of the built-up area, or the project is in an isolated location separated by substantial open space or sparsely settled area from the town or city–S = 0.

K.2: Away from Highways
The project cannot be located less than 200m away from a freeway or major arterial road.
Performance measure: distance from closest highway; if less than 200m–S = 0.

K.3: Healthful Location
Proximity of the site to any sources of pollution or harmful environmental impacts.
Performance measure: probability that the project will suffer negative environmental impacts (air, water, noise pollution, hazardous waste contamination, traffic hazards, etc.); if p = 1.0–S = 0.
C.1 Site location in relation to sources of pollution or other negative environmental impacts.
Performance measure: probability that the project will suffer negative environmental impacts (air, water, noise pollution, hazardous waste contamination, traffic hazards, etc.); $p_{min} = S_{max}$.

K.4: Link to Essential Facilities/Services
Inclusion in the project (see program) or adjacency to site of appropriate facilities for delivery of the following services:
Dining area/room and kitchen providing hot meals to residents; Multipurpose area for social activities, or appropriate rooms for specific social/cultural purposes; Office space for the administrator of the complex, located overlooking the main access; Laundry area or provision of laundry service for residents.
Performance measures: included–S = 1; not included–S = 0.
C.2 Services Accessibility (for any housing for relatively independent elderly)
Accessibility of the following facilities/services is scored on a range ac-

cording to criticality of the service. For the most critical services, $S_{max} = 5$; for the least critical, $S_{max} = 2$; S_{min} always $= 0$. Accessibility measures are: within or adjacent to project; accessible by foot; accessible by public transportation; not accessible.

Services (in order of criticality):
Grocery/food store; Pharmacy/drugstore; Religious facility (according to context: church, chapel, synagogue, etc.); Other stores/shopping; Barber/ hairdresser/beautician-cosmetics; Bank; Post Office; Library; Medical services; Public gardens or park; Senior day center; Community welfare/social services; Cafe or restaurant; Urban cultural amenities (museum, theatre, concert hall, etc.); Urban commercial/shopping center.

Site

K.5: Appropriate Land Use Designation
For congregate or sheltered housing or Type A (small) nursing homes: if the designated land use of the site is residential, $S = 1$; if it is other, $S = 0$. For Type B (large) nursing homes: if the designated land use of the site is residential or public/institutional, $S = 1$; if it is other, $S = 0$.
C.3 Secondary Land Uses
To what degree do any proposed secondary land uses on the site serve the needs of (a) the project residents; (b) neighborhood and/or city residents; or: to what degree are they inappropriate for the proposed housing and/or the character of the surrounding neighborhood? If no secondary land uses, S_{max}.

K.6: Size of Site
Is the area of the site equal to or larger than the area required by the prescribed Floor-area-ratio for the proposed project? Yes: $S = 1$; No: $S = 0$.
C.4 Relation Between Building Layout and Site Size and Configuration
Are the size and shape of the site appropriate for the proposed layout of building/s, and to what degree do they facilitate suitable development of exterior spaces and amenities?

K.7: Topography and Road System
Do the proposed on-site roads meet standard requirements (grades and turning radii)? Yes: $S = 1$; No: $S = 0$.

K.8: Pedestrian Path System
Does the topography enable pedestrian access on paths with grades not exceeding 5%, with minimal and selective use of ramps with grades not exceeding 1:12 (8.5%)? Yes: $S = 1$; No: $S = 0$.

C.5 Landform and Climate

To what extent do the site's landforms, combined with its microclimatic characteristics (orientation, shelter, prevailing winds, etc.) enable appropriate development of external spaces as sheltered and shaded areas for residents' seating and recreation?

C.6 Quality of Development and Landscaping

To what extent do the project's external development and landscaping enhance the following functions: easy pedestrian access to all appropriate areas; attractive gardens and landscaped areas; seating areas which are sheltered and accessible from residential buildings and common areas?

K.9: Access to Entrance

Does the plan provide appropriate access to the main entrance for pedestrians and vehicles? Yes: $S = 1$; No: $S = 0$.

C.7 Convenience of Access to Entrance

How convenient (close, unobstructed, noncircuitous, etc.) is access to the entrance from the nearest public road (a) for pedestrians; (b) for vehicles?

C.8 Site Bounding

To what extent does the project plan enable appropriate definition and bounding of the site into areas which are common to project and neighborhood residents, and private areas restricted to project residents only?

Building/Complex Layout

K.10: Minimum Size (for sheltered/congregate housing)

Does the project include at least 13 dwelling units? Yes: $S = 1$; No: $S = 0$.

C.9 Project Size

Scored according to optimum size criteria; e.g., 25-100 DUs: S_{max}, to Over 250 DUs: S_{min}.

C.10 Project Scale–Match Between Size and Environment

To what extent does the project's scale (size and layout) fit the character of its proximate environment and neighborhood?

K.11: Emergency Vehicle Access

Is reasonable access provided for emergency vehicles to all parts of the project and site that are accessible to and used by residents? Yes: $S = 1$; No: $S = 0$.

C.11 Vehicular Access and Road System

To what extent does the proposed road system provide convenient vehicular access for residents, staff, and visitors to appropriate entrances and parking, and easy access for emergency vehicles wherever necessary?

K.12: Adequate Parking

For congregate/sheltered housing:

Does the project provide (the maximum of) at least 1 parking space per 6 residential units OR the minimum parking required by the applicable local government regulation? Yes: S = 1; No: S = 0.

For nursing homes:

Does the project provide (the maximum of) at least 1 parking space per 6 residential units assigned to independent residents, OR the minimum parking required by the applicable local government regulation; AND parking spaces for residents of units/wards/wings assigned to frail and/or impaired elderly according to applicable standards set for hospitals? Yes: S = 1; No: S = 0.

C.12 Parking Convenience

To what extent does the project provide convenient parking for staff, resident, visitor, and emergency vehicles, with easy access between respective parking areas and the relevant entrances?

K.13: Match Between Building Layout and Environment

Does the layout of the proposed building/s (massing and height, site coverage, density and architectural character) contrast negatively with the character of the surrounding neighborhood and built environment? Yes: S = 0; No: S = 1.

C.13 Integration Between Proposed Housing and Neighborhood

To what extent is the layout and character of the proposed building/s integrated into the neighborhood and blends with its built environment?

K.14: Pavillions and Enclosed Walkways (this criterion reflects existing Israeli regulation): If the building layout is made up of separate pavillions or includes pavillions, are these linked by enclosed passages with a minimum width of 1.80m?

Buildings

C.14 Appearance–Integration in Neighborhood

To what extent is the external appearance of proposed buildings (form, external materials and roof, window treatments, balconies, architectural style, etc.) appropriate and integrated with the character of the surrounding neighborhood?

K.15: Conformity to Applicable Standards/Regulations

Are the buildings proposed in the project in compliance with the standards and regulations that apply to them (cite relevant statutes and applicable contingencies; e.g., in Israel, for congregate housing and nursing homes:

the applicable regulations of the Ministry of Labor and Welfare, and for Supportive Care Wards and any health-related facilities, the licencing procedures and standards of the Health Ministry), regarding room sizes and relations, materials, and equipment? Yes: $S = 1$; No: $S = 0$.

These evaluation criteria can be applied in the course of regulatory review of proposals for elderly housing, on the basis of information provided in the plans submitted for approval. In their more sophisticated version, the criteria can be combined into a systematic multi-criteria evaluation matrix, with appropriate weights assigned to the optional criteria (C1-14) to reflect their respective priority or importance.[12] In an alternative simplified application, this evaluation scheme can be used without weights or scoring, as a checklist for project assessment. It has been distributed as an advisory circular for use in plan review by local Planning and Building Commissions and District Planning and Building Commissions, and is being used for review of exceptional proposals that require assessment by the Planning Administration of the Interior Ministry.

NOTES

1. However, as will be detailed later, housing for the elderly in Israel is also subject to other regulations relating to its operation.

2. In the absence of criteria defining housing for the elderly, developers could obtain permission to build at higher densities by describing their projects as congregate housing for the elderly (see below). Evidence of such abuses prompted the Planning Administration of the Israel Ministry of the Interior to commission the report on which this paper is based (Alexander, 1994).

3. Consequently, the study's terms of reference are limited to planning criteria (which will be elaborated below), and do not include design criteria (e.g., internal building plans, room arrangements or sizes, building components such as stairs or ramps, equipment or fittings, etc.) or building and construction standards.

4. This will be addressed under regulative recommendations later.

5. The current regulations (Ministry of Labor and Welfare, 1986) define a "hostel" requiring a permit as any facility housing thirteen or more dependent elderly.

6. As the administrator of publicly-owned land (over 80% of all the land in Israel, and over 60% of all urban land), the Israel Land Administration is an active participant in the planning and development control system.

7. The only exception to this is the membership of a Ministry of Health official on the District Town Planning and Building Commissions, but this has had little practical impact.

8. This is a "floating" (i.e., locationally indeterminate) zone for proposals meeting certain landuse and size criteria, which substitutes a negotiated approval process for the rigid usage and density prescriptions of regular zoning.

9. Evidence for this are the frequent press accounts of malfeasance and mismanagement in nursing home operations, which often reach scandalous dimensions before coming to the attention of State regulatory agencies.

10. The Planning and Construction Ministry (*Bundesministerium für Raumordnung, Bauwesen und Städtebau*) and the Ministry for Family and Seniors.

11. Communication, C. Cornwell, Special Needs Housing branch, Department of the Environment, 22/2/1993.

12. For more on multi-criteria evaluation, see, e.g., Zeleny (1981) and Voogd (1983).

REFERENCES

Alexander, E.R. (1994) Evaluation Criteria for Plans of Housing for the Elderly. Jerusalem: Israel Ministry of the Interior, Planning Administration (Hebrew: Madadei Ha'aracha le'Tochniot Diur le'Zkenim).

Alexander, E.R., R. Alterman and H. Law-Yone (1983) *Evaluating Plan Implementation: The National Statutory Planning System in Israel.* Oxford: Pergamon.

Altman, I., M.F. Lawton and J.F. Wohlwill (eds.) (1984) *Elderly People and the Environment.* New York: Plenum Press.

Carstens, D.C. (1985) *Site Planning and Design for the Elderly: Issues, Guidelines and Alternatives.* New York: Van Nostrand-Reinhold.

Chellis, R.D., J.F. Seagle, Jr. and B.M. Seagle (1982) *Congregate Housing for Older People: A Solution for the 1980s.* Lexington, MA: Heath.

Cullingworth, J.B. (1993) *The Political Culture of Planning: American Land Use Planning in a Comparative Perspective.* New York/London: Routledge.

Department of the Environment (U.K.) (1974) Housing the Elderly. Lancaster: MTP Construction.

Faludi, A. and A. v.d. Valk (1994) *Rule and Order: Dutch Planning Doctrine in the Twentieth Century.* Dordrecht: Kluwer.

Federal Housing Administration (U.S.) (1966) Minimum Property Standards: Housing for the Elderly with special consideration for the Handicapped. Washington, DC: USGPO.

Hunt, M.E. (1991) "The Design of Supportive Environments for Older People." *Journal of Housing for the Elderly*, 9, 1/2: 127-140.

Israel Lands Authority (1991) Institutions for the Elderly: Program and Land Allocation. Jerusalem (Hebrew: Minhal Mekarkei Israel: Mosdot Lezkenim: Programma ve'Haktza'ot Karka).

Krupat, E. (1985) *People in Cities: The Urban Environment and Its Effects.* Cambridge: Cambridge University Press.

Lawton, M.P. (1986) *Environment and Aging* (2nd Ed.). Albany, NY: Center for the Study of Aging.

Marans, R.W., M.E. Hunt and K.L. Vakalo (1984) "Retirement Communities," (pp. 57-93) in Altman et al. (eds.) op. cit.

Ministry of Construction and Housing (Israel) (1991) Guidelines for Planning

Projects (1.52) Sheltered Housing for the Elderly–Summary of Requirements/ Checklist. Jerusalem (Hebrew: Misrad HaBinui VehaShikun: Hankhaiot le'Avodot Tikhnun (1.52) Diur LeKshishim–Rikuz Drishot/Rishimat Bakara).

Ministry of Health (Israel) (1991) Summary of Procedures Issued by the Division for Chronic Diseases and Aging. Jerusalem (Hebrew: Misrad HaBriut: Kovetz Nohalim Mita'am HaAgaf LeMakhalot Memushachot veZikna).

Ministry of Housing and Local Government (U.K.) (1969) Housing Standards and Costs: Accommodation Specially Designed for Old People. Circular 82/69, Whitehall, London.

Ministry of Labor and Welfare (Israel) (1986) Regulations for Inspection of Hostels: Maintenance of Independent and Frail Elderly in Hostel. Jerusalem (Hebrew: Misrad Ha'Avoda Ve'Revakha: Takanot Le'Pikuakh al haMe'onot–Achzakat Zkenim Atzmaiim Ve'Tshushim beMeonot).

Monk, A. and L.W. Kaye (1991) "Congregate Housing for the Elderly: Its Need, Function and Perspectives." *Journal of Housing for the Elderly*, 9, 1/2: 5-19.

Regnier, V. and J. Pynoos (1987) *Housing the Aged: Design Directives and Policy Considerations.* New York/Amsterdam: Elsevier.

Valins, M. (1982) *Housing for Elderly People: A Guide for Architects, Interior Designers and Their Clients.*

Voogd, H. (1983) *Multiple Criteria Evaluation for Urban and Regional Planning.* London: Pion.

Zeleny, M. (1981) *Multiple Criteria Decision Making.* New York: McGraw-Hill.

Index

T - #0555 - 101024 - C0 - 212/152/10 - PB - 9780789013309 - Gloss Lamination